THE SNACK BOX DIET

A TOTALLY NEW WAY TO LOSE FAT AND GET FIT

Mark Moxom

ISBN 978-0-9582931-1-2

Notice

This book is intended as a reference volume only and in no way should be construed as a medical manual. The contents are intended to help you understand and make informed decisions about your health and fitness and so should never be considered as a replacement for treatment you have been given by your medical advisor or fitness professional. You must seek competent medical advice if you suspect you have a medical condition no matter how small.

The publisher or author assumes no responsibility or liability for damage to you or any other person arising from the use of any product, information, instruction or idea contained in the contents or through the use of services mentioned in this book. Use of this material is solely at the readers risk.

To Willow

"You don't make progress by standing on the sidelines, whimpering and complaining. You make progress by implementing ideas."

Shirley Hu

CONTENTS

1. BEFORE YOU DO ANYTHING

When people see old photos of a very fat me, they often can't believe it's the same person. The fat loss has been drastic. Over the years, I passed on the things that I learnt about fat loss to others about what works and what doesn't and so on and on many occasions people have said to me that I should write a book about it.

Frankly, the seeds of this diet have been in my mind for years. Over that time I've made careful notes of all the many things I wanted to include. Yet each time I sat down to read through it, I wasn't satisfied with everything I had written down- there was too much information. All good solid information but just too much. So I started to simplify things as much as I could.

It was clear that most people aren't going to be too concerned about all the reasoning behind the diet. They just want a diet that works, is easy to follow and doesn't leave them hungry.

So that's exactly what I've put in the book!

I've taken out a lot of the stuff that initially was going to go into the book - all the reasons why things work, the detailed social and cultural aspects of fat loss, many do's and don'ts and so much more. Leaving in place just the things you really need to know and must do in order to get fit and lose fat successfully.

So the book that we have ended up with isn't just a "what to do book" neither is it a "why you should do it book" (although parts of both of those things are in there) It is very much a "how to do it book"

You simply have to follow the instructions - connect the dots if you like - in order to get the results you want.

I'm an engineer. Not a doctor or dietician. Simply an engineer who loves food (and cooking) so much I could easily get as fat as a pig. In fact I did get as fat as a pig which was why I needed to diet.

I tried lots of ways to lose the fat and get fit and sadly most of them had only partial success and none of them really helped with my limited will power or satisfied my hunger totally.

In the end, I put my 'engineers' cap on and tackled getting fit and slim like an engineer would. I took all the good bits from those diets that worked for me a little and refined and honed them into a diet that worked for me completely. One that overcame the desire to snack, the hunger from not eating enough and so on - but caused me to lose the fat, get fit and healthy again.

Here is the solution. And I'm happy to call it THE solution because it works.

The Snack Box Diet is simple to do, effective, healthy and overcomes the failings of other diets. It will help you to get slim, fit, and active without having to suffer hunger, guilt or failure.

There's no calorie counting, no portions to juggle or any real messing about. Simply make up your snack box and your set for the day.

2. QUICK START GUIDE

Right now, you just might want to get on with it so here is the quick way to get started. In eight easy steps.

1. Go to Part Two and find the shopping list for week one.

2. See what you need to buy and go and get it.

If you don't have one already - you will need a snack box.

Any sealable plastic box will do - I use two - One about 9"x5"x3½" or 22x13x9 cm and a smaller one for the dish of the day that's about 5"x3"x2" or 13x8x5 cm. Also a small sealable jar to carry the dressings and so on.

3. Empty the house of temptations

4. Measure yourself and mark down those measurement on the chart at the back of the book in the 'Progress Logs' chapter

5. Prepare your first snack box for the next day

6. Go through the next day eating only what you have put in the snack box.

7. Make up your box for the next day (it's OK to snack while your doing it – but ONLY on food items from the OK list)

Congratulations, you have just completed your first day on

the snack box diet.

8. Now go through the rest of the book paying particular attention to the chapters called...

There is No Need to Fail

What You Can Eat - The List of OK Foods

Starting The Diet

Measuring Your Progress

And doing the 'Brain Work' in Part Two

By the way. You don't have to wait until a Monday to start the diet. It's not the day that matters - it's the starting.

3. HOW DOES THE DIET WORK?

The short answer is that it works with the body and overcomes the many problems that previous diets could not deal with.

If you've tried any other diet before then you can probably testify that...

- They left you hungry
- That basically the food you were eating did not satisfy you
- They did not help you deal with those peckish times throughout the day
- There was not enough variety of food to eat
- They gave you no real incentive to carry on

The fact of the matter is this... We have put on fat because it"s too easy to eat too much of the wrong types of food instead of eating the foods our bodies need. But it's not all our fault! Because through the example of those around us, advertising, and many other reasons - we are encouraged to eat far too much food.

How many times have you gone away from the table patting your stomach with that false pained look on your face and said to anyone who is listening "oh, I've eaten far too much"?

Not only that. Most modern diets, have fallen for the falsehood that fats are bad for you and consequently restrict the amount of fat that you are able to eat. That means that they very quickly cut out red meats, (or any 'fatty' meats), cheese and other milk products or anything that is considered to have a high measure of fat in it.

They then proceed to replace those fats with the only things that they have left which are things like potatoes, pasta, rice, bread and every other kind of food that has a high glycemic value and often a very high carbohydrate content.

The problem with that is that carbohydrates are very quickly metabolised by the body so no sooner have you eaten them - you start to feel hungry again.

Other diets also like to limit the amount of food that you eat which means you have the double whammy of having even less of the food that does not satisfy your body in the first place.

But to compound the problems of these types of diet, you are also encouraged to eat only at certain times of the day and never between meals.

The Snack Box Diet overcomes the problems of traditional diets quite easily because of what you are encouraged to eat and how you are encouraged to eat it.

Firstly, the food you are encouraged to eat has a higher protein and fat content than many other diets. That's because it's a scientific fact that protein and fat rich foods take longer to be digested. This in turn means that the body finds those types of food more satisfying. In a nutshell, that means you don't get hungry as quickly as you would normally do on say a calorie restricted diet.

Secondly, the amount of these foods that you can eat on the Snack Box Diet are "within reason" not restricted. Neither are you encouraged to eat only at certain times in fact, you are encouraged to eat "when you are peckish" before hunger has a chance to take hold.

So in a nutshell, the Snack Box Diet encourages you to eat nutritious food that your body finds satisfying - just when your body needs it.

Thirdly, because your not binging on food, you are allowing your stomach to return to its normal, natural size. This in turn means that you become increasingly satisfied with steadily decreasing quantities of food.

All in all, it is these three factors that make the snack box diet so effective.

Which leads me to another point.

Because your giving your body food to which it is better suited, your body will use that food much more efficiently. That means that your body will start to 'demand' gradually decreasing quantities of food. You will not have to force a calorie restrictive diet on your body – it will - of it's own accord – be doing that for it's self.

You will be hard pushed to find a better or simpler way of helping your body get in shape than this one.

Another thing that most diets over look is that we are not just a body wandering around looking for food to eat.

We have, thoughts, emotions, ideals, needs, wants, desires, relationships, pressures and many other things that shape and make up the person we are. And much of the time these 'parts' of who we are, aren't necessarily working together

Unless these other parts are also taken into account and understood - then it does not matter how nutritionally brilliant a diet is - it won't be effective because not every part of who we are is behind getting the body is shape.

Once again, the Snack Box Diet gives you the tools you need in order to get every part of you 'on side' so that everything that makes you, you - all of the complicated parts of your being - become dedicated to getting your body in shape.

4. THERE IS NO NEED TO FAIL

Many people fail to finish a diet for one simple reason and one simple reason alone.

They don't really know why they are dieting!

Now that may surprise you after all common sense does tell us that nobody would start something that is not going to be easy, without knowing why they're doing it. But the fact of the matter is, is that many people do start dieting with only the vaguest of notions of why they're doing it in the first place.

Let us have a very quick look at what some of those vague reasons might be ...

- I've got too fat
- I'm overweight
- I need to get fit
- My Clothes don't fit me any more
- My husband/wife says I'm a little chubby

And many more like these ...

Now while these may be statements of fact - that does not make them reasons - at least not sufficiently good enough reasons to inspire us to see a diet through to the very end.

Just as getting out of condition and gaining fat was something that change the way you are i.e. something that changed your life and obviously not for the better. Then reversing that, getting fit and fat free is also something that is life changing and it needs a life changing reason in order for you to be able to carry it through.

So what is a life changing reason?

Let's take an easy one to start with.

If your doctor tells you that you are morbidly overweight and unless you lose forty pounds - you are in line for a heart attack. Then that's a life changing reason.

If you find you can't play with your children or grandchildren like you would like to because you're so out of condition, but know that you could do if you only got fit and lost the fat. Then that's a life changing reason

If you know that your being overweight is causing you to miss out on that well-deserved promotion (and believe me it really does). Then getting rid of that barrier to your success is indeed a life changing reason.

In fact, if being out of condition and overweight is stopping you from enjoying any part of your life or is holding you back in any way - then dealing with it can only be a life changing experience.

The bottom line is this. Finding a real reason - or reasons - for getting fit and losing the fat - will be the thing that carries you through those times when you'll be wondering "is it really worth it".

But find out what is the real reason why you want to get fit and fat free?

Strangely enough, you just have to ask someone who knows.

Blankly, you need to ask yourself - and not be satisfied with glib answers or reasons you have heard other people give. You have to dig deeper into who you are and find out what are the real and deep seated reasons for why you want to change and why you got fat in the first place.

That, for some people may not be an easy task. So for that reason I'm going to help you by giving you the simple tools you need to make that process easier.

So, what we are going to do now is use the lined pages (Which you'll find in part 2) to write down your lists.

The first list is of all the negative things - it's a list of those things that being overweight and under fit stopped you from doing.

Let me give you a few to be going on with ...

- I can't run around with the children/grandchildren
- I can't go to the beach because people laugh at me
- I can't take the dog for a walk, it's just too exhausting
- I can't wear my favourite clothes any more
- I have so little energy
- My love life isn't as good as it used to be

So now take a pen and write down everything - and I mean everything that you can think of - that being overweight is causing you to miss out on.

Turn to Part two of the book where you'll find a place for you to fill in all the things you can think of...

Come back here when you have finished doing that.

11

Why are you Fat?

So by now you will have written down all the things that being overweight is stopping you from doing or achieving.

One thing I have learnt over the years of helping people get fit and lose fat is that very often being overweight is actually a symptom of something not being right somewhere else in their life.

Quite often, people turn to food as a way to take their minds off of other things going on in their lives that they're not comfortable with.

Everything in life has a cause and effect. So if there is something in your life that is causing you grief - getting rid of the cause of that problem will make dealing with the symptoms of the problem (getting fat) so much easier.

That's why the next list that you're going to write out is even more powerful one than the one that you've already written down. This is a list of your needs, wants and desires.

Simply put, if you can identify your needs wants and desires you get the double effect of firstly, finding out what is missing from your life and secondly, you give yourself something to aim for.

This is an important step - don't be tempted to avoid it.

It's really very simple. All you need to do is write down everything that you want in and from your life. This is your wish list, this is a list of everything you would like to accomplish in your life, everything you'd like to have whether it's a physical thing, a personal quality or trait or whatever.

What we're trying to do here is help you to get to know yourself better- get to know the real you - the person you would really like to be if there was nothing slowing you down or stopping you.

This is an important step because - as you go through your wish list - you may well find that one thing, that one special reason that will carry you through when everything else seems to be meaningless.

Now to make it easy for you I've broken this task down into three parts and also included a few suggestions for each part.

The lists are...

- List Number One - The Things I Feel I Need Right Now
- List Number Two - The Things I Want
- List Number Three - Personal Qualities I Want and Need

Out of the three, obviously one and two will be the easiest for you to do simply because they deal with physical or tangible things. List three however may seem a little bit more difficult.

Firstly, because we have a tendency to think that we are already perfect. Secondly, because it's something that we rarely ever think about. And thirdly, because it's in our nature to make do with what we have and settle for second best.

That is an unconscious admission that we think we are not worth any better. Frankly, I think you are worthy of having the best of everything and I hope that you will too.

But don't worry about it. Use the examples I've given you as a starting point and see where you get to from there.

List Number One - The Things I Feel I Need Right Now

Some suggestions:

1. All my bills totally paid
2. Being fit enough to walk the dog or to do ??...
3. Enough money to pay my rent or mortgage and general day-to-day expenses
4. Having the energy to play with the children/ grandchildren
5. Enough income to afford the holiday that I really need to take
6. Being healthy enough to give up the medication I am taking

So these are just a few suggestions. But really, don't be worried because your putting everything you need down on this list - just do it. Whatever you do, don't start limiting yourself - put everything down - even those things you may not feel comfortable admitting that you need.

So once again, turn to List Number One in part two of this book

List number two That - The Things I Want

Now this is not a list of things that you need, it's a list of the things that you want to have whether you need them or not. Again, don't limit yourself in any way as the saying goes "the sky is the limit"

Some suggestions:

1. Excellent health
2. A million in the bank
3. A comfortable house
4. Be super fit - Describe in detail the body you want!
5. A happy home life
6. Brilliant holidays in fantastic places
7. Canoeing down the Amazon
8. A holiday home in Barbados.

This time, turn to List Number Two in part two of this book.

List Number Three - Personal Qualities I Want and Need

Thinking about it, it's obvious that you are going to want more out of life than mere things so here's your chance to include the things that you think are important for a successful, high quality life.

If you look at the lives of any successful people you'll notice that they possess certain qualities or attributes of both personality and character. Many times we do actually possess those qualities and attributes ourselves, but they remain hidden. And sometimes another persona emerges instead of the real us.

I think the list of suggestions will actually help to explain this more readily.

Some Suggestions:

1.   Be more disciplined
2.   Be in good health
3.   Have a better disposition
4.   Be friendlier to others
5.   The enthusiastic
6.   Be more assertive
7.   Have real self-confidence

This time, turn to List Number Three in part two of this book

5. DON'T COMPARE YOURSELF TO OTHERS

The fact that this diet treats you as a unique person means that you never have any need to compare yourselves unfavourably with others.

There are actually only three people who matter as far as this diet is concerned. They are ...

1. The person you were at the start of the diet

2. The person you are now

3. The person you want to be at the end of the diet.

And as all of them are you - that puts you in complete control.

You have no need to keep up with the Joneses (unless you are a Jones of course) and certainly will never be asked to compare yourself with anybody else even if they're doing the same diet.

You have the body you have now because a unique set of circumstances worked to make it the way it is.

In the main these circumstances will have been influenced and controlled by things like your country of origin, ethnicity, where you live now, who your parents were, who you married, and more.

Let's takes some of those in turn and see how they affect who we are.

Where you come from...

Many in the diet, health and fitness world shy away from the subject of ethnicity, it's almost as if they're frightened to be labelled as racist. But the fact of the matter is, is that these thing play an important part in giving you the body you have now. And it is certain you can't escape from your genes - they have made you the person that you are.

Our ethnic origins are a big part of that and so they have to be dealt with in a rational manner.

Where you come from can and does obviously affect the how's and whys of the body shape that you now have. Even more so where there has been a change in what you eat.

It goes without saying that people from different regions of the world are going to have different diets. That is a straight forward fact.

But even if you stick in one region another fact is that diets both national and regional - change over time - no matter what country you look at.

For instance, the diet of a typical rural western teenager today is full of processed foods high in sugars, starches, fillers and preservatives. And most likely - sadly lacking in good quality fresh vegetables and additive free meat.

If you compare that to the diet that their grandparents would have eaten back in say the 50s - you will see that there are huge differences. First in terms of the quantity of food eaten and secondly in the actual make up of the ingredients that food contained.

The grandparents food would be significantly lower in processed ingredients and at the same time higher in things such as fresh vegetables and other wholesome ingredients.

And frankly, it doesn't matter what country you look at (where obesity is becoming a problem) you will find a similar pattern emerging in that the diet has changed for the worse.

Where countries have become more influenced by Western culture these changes can appear to be even more radical - particularly where local foods have been pushed aside by the so-called convenience of fast foods.

Here's a little anecdote that illustrates that...

Some years ago, I would occasionally eat in a cafe serving kebabs, falafel's and that sort of food. One day there were two new members of staff who started working there. They were Kurdish refugees who had escaped the problems in their own country to make a new life for themselves. These young men were hard working, conscientious and always happy to exchange friendly banter with the customers. Now, I often used to be in their when it was quiet which gave us the opportunity to chat with each other about all sorts of things and one day we got onto the subject of food.

Like I said, the food they were serving in the cafe was kebabs, falafel's so I asked one of the guys if that was the type of food they ate at home.

They said "no". While you might find that sort of food in the towns back in the old country, the food eaten at home consisted of things like bulghur wheat, fruit and vegetables (lots of cucumbers apparently) and so on. Meat was only eaten on special occasions. One of the things they found most surprising when they first came into the country was simply the huge variety of food that was available. What shocked them even more was the amount of food people would eat.

Over about the space of six months I noticed that these fit young men were starting to develop what can only be described as a little bit of a paunch. Me being me, I reminded them of the conversation we had previously about how they found the food when they first came here - and pointing to their new-found girth - said that they had obviously taken a liking to the food they were getting here.

They both agreed that while they were working just as hard if not harder than they used to work back at home, they were also eating a lot more than they used to eat. And they both confessed to eating a lot more bread and cakes than they ever had done before.

It's a nice little story that serves to illustrate a number of things about how a change in circumstance or location can so easily affect our bodies and health.

All without us noticing!

Adopted Dishes

Over the last 30 or 40 years foreign travel has opened up many opportunities for us to try food that we would not normally have tried. At the same time, the mobilisation of world population has meant that people from differing cultural, ethnic, and culinary backgrounds have – as they moved in from different countries - all brought with them a real rich diversity of differing dishes. These have been gradually adopted by the population of the countries that they've come to be part of.

In the US, there has been a distinct rise in the influence of Spanish, Chinese and Indian culinary arts. The United Kingdom has seen a distinct rise in Indian, Chinese and African dishes becoming better known. Australia and New Zealand have also seen their culinary tastes changed and influenced by the many people who have come from far and wide who have made that country their home.

And frankly, our culinary heritage has been enriched by them doing so, and at the same time these incomes have been exposed to new types of food in their countries of adoption.

Yet another example of a change in diet.

Who Your Parents Are

Our parents are probably the most significant influence in our likes and dislikes as far as food goes. In fact it is enshrined in our culture with sayings like "just like your mother used to make", "home-made" and many more I'm sure you can think of.

As a general rule, we will all continue eating the type of foods that we used to eat with our parents. If our parents used to supply good wholesome healthy food, though most of the time we will continue to eat good wholesome healthy food. At the other end of the scale, if the most used item in the kitchen was a microwave - then we will probably continue in the same manner.

I suppose the extreme would be if every meal consisted of home delivered pizzas or Chinese or something like that, then you will probably find that same pattern continuing in the next generation.

Who You Married

It's an old saying "the way to a man's heart is through his stomach" unfortunately the modern reality of that has missed out one word "attack" and the new version of that saying reads "the way to a man's heart attack is through his stomach"

Seriously though, getting married or certainly getting into a serious relationship is the type of occasion that promotes one of the greatest changes in what we eat.

For men as much as women the change can be quite significant. Once we get settled down there is also a tendency to become complacent and not take the same amount of care about ourselves as we did when we were single. I'll bet you can name at least one friend who has put on the pounds after tying the knot.

Your Children's Influence

You can't get away from the fact that children love to be part of the in crowd and that means if the in crowd all eat at McD's or all have a certain type of pizza - then your children will want to be exactly the same as them

The problem arises when the influence of your children's friends on what they eat starts to limit what they 'will' eat and even worse, what they're willing to try.

When I was young, I was very finicky eater as well. In fact for a number of years the only things I would eat were cornflakes with lots of milk and sugar, french fries and things like toast. This obviously drove my mother to distraction.

After this had gone on for a fair while she took me off to the doctors to see if there was anything wrong with me as I wasn't eating properly no matter how much she insisted.

He was an old-fashioned, wise doctor and his response was "for the moment it doesn't seem to be doing any harm - so there's no point worrying about it as I'm sure he'll grow out of it"

And sure enough I did - eventually!

But the thing is, I got into the habit of eating a very limited range of foods which led to a habit of never thinking about trying new foods and new dishes. Sadly, it wasn't until my 20s that this habit was broken.

I'd got into a culinary rut so deep - I could not see there were other things I could try and maybe enjoy.

When I look back upon my childhood I do regret some of the wonderful food that I missed out on simply because I wasn't willing to try it. And I wonder too, if some of the usual childhood illnesses I suffered may not have been lessened or avoided if I'd have eaten better in those formative years.

When my son was little he, like most kids, went through the stage of not "liking" foods that he had quite happily eaten a few days beforehand.

One day, he uttered the fateful words "I don't like it, I've never tried it" and I realised I was staring at a mini me.

I didn't want him to go through the same things that I had gone through and miss out as much as I had missed out just through being unwilling to try things. So I asked him "how can you know you don't like it if you've never tried it?" After a few moments reflection he looked up and said "I don't know"

So I explained to him my story and told him I didn't want him to miss out on all the things that I'd missed out on, but I would never insist that he ate anything providing he could tell me why he didn't like it. We agreed that he would always try things if I asked him to and if he didn't like it, well that was OK, he didn't have to eat it.

And try them he did!

Obviously, he didn't like everything as children, like adults, do have things they like and dislike - but he was always willing to try. And so thankfully didn't have the limited diet that I had

23

through my teenage years.

But what we eat is not the only thing that matters in forming the body we have. Obviously, things like our lifestyle, our age, the job we do and so much more also has a profound affect on out physical being.

Over the last 30 or 40 years jobs have become far less physically demanding.

When I was young I had a job on a building site. On my first day on the job, we had to unload a delivery lorry by hand. It was carrying 15 tons of 1 CWT (about 50 kg) bags of cement. Not too difficult I thought until I realised the driver was throwing them on to our shoulders two at a time.

Today, that same job would be done by a forklift or hoist on the delivery truck itself.

In virtually every sector of commerce, the amount of physical effort required to do a job has been lessened or removed entirely.

The same is true in many homes as well with modern appliances taking on the physical drudge of housework. But a lack of natural exercise opportunities is not just limited to adults.

Kids today don't go out side to play as my friends and I did back in the 60's and 70's. They are far more likely to be found in front of the TV or computer instead.

The point is we just don't move around as much as we did in previous generations. But at the same time, we eat far more than our parents and grand parents did so it's no wonder that 'we' are getting fat.

Exercise in some form or another is missing and needs to be put back into our daily lives.

6. EXERCISE - NOT AN OPTION

People often ask "is exercise an option - do I really have to do it?"

I think the first thing to overcome is a preconception that people have about exercise. It's true to say that when you mention the word exercise - many people think about having to go to a gym, maybe running or jogging or getting involved with something along those sorts of lines.

But the point is that in reality getting more exercise really means increasing the amount of physical movement that your body gets to a level that is a bit more than what it is used to doing now.

Taking that 'bit more' to the extreme - could mean hiding the TV remote so that a couch potato would have to walk backwards and forwards to the television instead of using the remote.

Seriously though, increasing the amount of exercise that you get does not necessarily mean you need to join a gym or do anything like that.

For you, getting more exercise could just mean...

- Taking the dog for a walk each day.

- Going out dancing once or twice a week.

- Taking up yoga or tai chi

- Or if you're feeling a little bit energetic something like judo.

But the point I'm trying to make here is that yes, increasing the amount of exercise you do is necessary. But it's the "increase" that's important rather than the activity itself - at least initially.

You don't need a leotard

One excuse I have heard from some people is along the lines of 'I don't look good in a leotard'.

Quite frankly, I don't look good in a leotard either.

Let me say this very clearly. "You don't gain anything from the exercise you're doing by wearing a leotard."

Leotards are a fashion accessory! They are not necessary in order to exercise. The fact that most other people might be wearing them to do the particular form of exercise you are thinking of doing, doesn't mean to say that you have to follow suit. Neither does it mean that those leotard wearers are any better at what they are doing then you can be.

The only thing a leotard says about the wearer is that they are a slave to fashion. The bottom line - as far as what you wear for exercise is simple.

Wear something that you feel comfortable in and that is appropriate for the activity you are doing.

It really doesn't matter if that turns out to be a baggy T-shirt and tracksuit bottoms or whatever - it is entirely your choice. I'm sure you would not let yourself be dictated to about what you wear out on the street - so within reason, don't be dictated to by others about what you wear in the gym.

Providing what you wear is fresh, clean and appropriate - no right thinking person should take offense at your wearing something different from them.

And honestly, if the instructor or anybody else involved in running the facility insists you should wear a leotard - then they are more concerned about how they look to others than they are concerned about your health.

If that's the case leave - and find somewhere better.

What Exercise should I do?

When it comes to exercise, one of the many mistakes that a lot of people make is the choice of exercise regime that they go for.

In the heat and excitement of the great "new idea" to exercise, it's common for people to look around and see what others are doing. They then base their choice of exercise on the needs or wants and aspirations of those around them - instead of looking at their own needs, wants and aspirations.

This of course can only lead to disappointment later on, as sooner or later it will become apparent that the choice they made isn't really right for them.

It has to be remembered, that exercise for someone who is overweight, is not normally going to be a natural part of who they are at the moment. So any exercise regime they want to take up has to be something that they can incorporate into their daily routine so that when the first flush of excitement wears off it will not become too much of a chore to continue.

That's why it is imperative that any exercise regime that you decide to embark upon is one that you can comfortably continue with after the excitement has worn off and - equally importantly - when you have got the body that you desire.

It really is no use taking out a subscription to the smartest

27

gym in town if you're only going to use it half a dozen times.

You can exercise just as well without going to a gym as we shall see later on.

Exercise Buddy

Of course, having someone to exercise with is a great motivational tool. But choosing who you decide to exercise with is something that should also be done with considerable care. You need to find someone who is as committed as you are to exercising (or maybe even more committed than you are). Someone whom you know you can count on to be reliable and not prone to be easily distracted by such things as family life, their job or anything else that may provide a handy excuse.

There are basically two types of people that you should look for as an exercise buddy.

The first is someone who already exercises in the way that you know would be ideal for you and, has been doing so regularly for at least a year.

Ideally, they will have a similar lifestyle and commitment level as yourself. That way, you will know that they are able to deal with the day-to-day circumstances that will "endeavour" to interfere with your getting your necessary exercise.

The second type of person, is someone who may not yet have started exercising but who has the same level of 'need' to do as it yourself. And who also demonstrates in their own life real dedication and commitment to finish things they started.

Exercise Schedule

The next thing that needs to be sorted out is your exercise schedule. Ideally, this should be at a time on the same days every week that is the least likely to be interfered with by other things going on in your life.

If your life revolves mainly around your kids - then a mutually convenient time during school hours could be the ideal time slot for you and your exercise buddy.

Probably the best time to do that is after you've dropped them off at school. That's because - generally speaking - we tend to drop our children off at school at the same time every school day and because you're already out of the house, that's one less piece of inertia to try and overcome.

And remember too, that it doesn't have to be a mad rush to try and fit into the morning. In reality, if getting fit is important to you, then as much as you can, you should plan your day around your exercise.

And, if you're going to a gym, then why not take advantage of the other facilities that they have a treat yourself to a sauna or some other form of pampering. Maybe not every time - but at least once a week. Exercise, does not have to be a chore - it can and should be a pleasure. If it's not, you're doing the wrong sort of exercise for you.

On the other hand, if you're trying to fit exercise in and around regular work hours then quite often a little bit of lateral thinking can work wonders.

Many companies nowadays have gyms on the premises so the sensible option would be to make use of that. It's quite common for people to use the gym at lunchtime or after working hours and some even get in early to make use of the facilities. An other advantage is that these facilities are often free or exceptionally cheap to use. And even if your company doesn't have its own gym you will often find that there are very good gyms in and around working districts in many towns.

But this is where we come to use a little lateral thinking.

You are not necessarily limited to using the gym outside

working hours. If you can take advantage of flexitime then you might be to use the gym when everybody else is sat behind a desk. Quite often, this can mean flexing maybe just half an hour in order to take advantage of a quieter time in the gym.

For instance, if you can see that the gym is very busy between say 12 and 1pm - getting there at 11:30 would mean that you get the exercise you need without having to deal with the crowds. You might also find going a little later - after the midday session - will have the same effect. i.e. Everyone else is leaving just as you arrive. The point is, is to use your imagination and be flexible in order to make the best use of the facilities that you have available.

It's important to make sure that what ever exercise you decide upon is indeed a pleasure and not a chore. A little bit of forward planning can really help to make exercising something to look forward to rather than something to dread.

I've used going to the gym as the example in this case, but of course that's not the only type of exercise that you can get. There are a whole number of physical activities that you can involve yourself in that will provide you with the exercise that you need.

You might enjoy something like five aside football, or squash, table tennis, cycling, fencing or in fact anything that may loosely be regarded as a sport - provided it gives you enough exercise.

Other Forms of Exercise

But of course you're not limited to those things that may be regarded as sporting activities. Things like yoga, tai chi, Pilates and more can offer a sufficient level of exercise to meet the needs of many.

And again, something like dancing can offer a huge benefits

in terms of exercise - particularly with the more energetic forms of dance such as salsa, jive and le Roc. In addition, there is a huge social benefit that can be derived from dancing - plus of course you get the pleasure of learning new skills.

Activities like these also have the benefit of being held regularly throughout the week and would be ideally suited to those people who would prefer to get their "exercise" during the evening.

Again, if you choose to go down the social exercise route it's important to find something that you enjoy. And don't be put off by thinking that you need a partner either as there will normally be plenty of people - also going there on their own - for you to dance with.

So there you have it!

Exercise does not have to be a chore and in fact you should do your best to make sure it is not so - but rather is considered by you to be a real pleasure. Once you've decided on what form of exercise is best for you, make sure you incorporated into your weekly routine at a time that makes the most sense of what you are already doing.

The easier you make it to exercise the less excuses you have to avoid it, but more importantly, the more pleasure you will get from it.

Rather than just leave wondering what you can do. I have included a few basic exercises in part two in a chapter called 'A few Easy Exercises'. Turn to that when you' re ready to start...

Do I Need to See my Doctor Before I Start Exercising?

The short answer to that is probably no, but the sensible answer will have to be yes - particularly if you think that there is any chance that exercise could put your health at risk.

Take note however that thoughts of that nature are not an excuse for you to rule out exercise in any way. The fact is that no matter what state you are in physically - there is still some form of exercise that you can join in with.

To a certain extent, whether or not you go and see your doctor will depend on what type of exercise you decide to embark upon. For instance, if you are deciding to go and join a gym then the professionals involved in your signing up process would very quickly determine whether or not they thought it advisable for you to consult with your doctor or not before you started exercising.

Properly trained sports consultants are not stupid and if they had the slightest doubt about your capabilities they would soon tell you to go and see a doctor before you started exercising.

In fact the same could be said for any type of physical activity where you are in contact with a trainer, teacher or other professional

At that sort of level, the enrolment or acceptance procedures are usually designed to highlight those cases where a visit to the doctor would be advisable.

Obviously, where your chosen physical exercise does not involve a professional of that calibre, then you should take it upon yourself to go and see your doctor beforehand - if you have any doubts about your own physical capabilities.

Again, don't allow those doubts to dissuade you from embarking on something that will increase your level of physical activity. Just make sure you follow a sensible course of action that puts your own well-being first.

All this talk about exercise may have made you a bit peckish. So let's turn our attention to what we can eat on the Snack Box Diet.

7. WHAT YOU CAN EAT
THE LIST OF OK FOODS

You can probably eat a lot more than you thought you were going to be able to.

Meat Products.

You can eat all meats and poultry.

But do try and avoid those that are highly processed and may contain lots of fillers and additives

Fish Products

You can eat all fish.

And that includes fresh, frozen and tinned.

Dairy

You can eat all cheeses.

But note that he more processed cheese is the more likely it is to contain fillers and additives - these types of cheeses are therefore best avoided.

Milk and Cream

But not the low fat kind.

Vegetables you can eat

Artichoke	Onions
Aubergine	Pumpkin
Asparagus	Rhubarb
Avocado	Sauerkraut
Broccoli	Spaghetti squash
Brussels sprouts	Spring onions
Cauliflower	Sprouting broccoli
Courgettes	String Beans
Green beans	Turnips
Mange tout	Water Chestnuts

Salad ingredients you can eat

Alfalfa sprouts	Kale
Bean sprouts	Leeks
Bok Choi	Lettuce
Cabbage	Mushrooms
Celery	Mustard greens
Chicory	Okra
Chinese cabbage	Peppers
Chives	Radishes
Cucumber	Rocket
Endives	Sorrel
Escarole	Spinach
Fennel	Swiss chard
Jicama	Watercress

Nuts and Seeds You Can Eat

Armand's

Brazil nuts

Coconut

Hazelnuts

Pecans

Pine nuts

Pumpkin seeds

Sesame seeds

Sunflower seeds

Walnuts

Fats you can eat

All animal fats including butter and lard

Olive oil

Safflower oil

Sesame oil

Sunflower oil

Walnut oil

Peanut oil

Sweeteners (instead of sugar)

Stevia

Honey (used sparingly)

Herbs and Spices

These can be used as required.

What you cannot eat

Basically, if it's not on the above list then don't eat it - even in small portions.

Ideally, you want to stay away from all potatoes and most root vegetables, pasta, rice, bread or anything else that contains flour. You might have noticed that the 'don't eat list' is a list of foods high in carbohydrates and has a high glycemic index.

If something you fancy contains carbohydrates in any great quantity i.e above 5g per serving - then don't include it in your diet.

That's simply because you will get enough carbohydrates in what you eat throughout the day.

Even though you are encouraged to avoid foods that have fillers and additives, the fact of the matter it is that it's almost impossible to do so unless you are growing everything yourself.

So you will get quite a significant amount of carbohydrates hidden amongst what you are eating during the day.

8. HOW MUCH SHOULD I EAT?

How much you should eat depends on how big you are.

This is something you probably won't hear anywhere else but the simple fact is, is that the bigger your body is the more food it needs.

Most diets try to limit you to a predefined amount of food - most often determined by the amount of calories it contains.

However, that amount of calories is normally worked out for somebody who has an ideal body size.

It seems like no one has stopped to think or take notice of the obvious fact which is that - someone who wants to get fit and lose fat is normally going to be bigger than the average body size and a bigger body needs more energy to move around.

Taking that into account, the quantity of food suggested for this diet has been worked out for someone who is about twenty pounds overweight. This is just a starting point. If you find that you have too much food then cut it down.

If, on the other hand you find that there is not enough food add a little more.

Best practice would be to add more from the meat, salad

and vegetable selection. But do so sensibly.

No matter how well any diet has been designed you can't move away from the fact that if you are eating more food than your body needs in order to function - it will turn a lot of the excess food into fat - and that's not what you want.

9. STARTING THE DIET

Following this diet is incredibly easy as there is no counting calories and (within reason) no restrictions on the quantity of permitted food that you can eat. In fact, you can eat freely from the snack box throughout the day and ideally you will have put enough in it to last you the whole day. But even if you haven't, then you can refill it with any of the top up foods on the OK list so that you'll never go hungry.

So let's get started ...

Clear the house of Temptation

If you're like me then there are many things that can tempt you and sometimes it just seems easier to give in.

I've found one of the most effective ways of getting over that problem is simply to get everything that can cause big temptation out of the house. Now obviously that is a lot easier the fewer people there are in the house. But even if you are in the midst of a family then there's still a lot you can do.

Now if chocolate is your thing then, assuming that the kids

are old enough, why not get them to keep it in their own room. Simply tell them that you're on a new diet and you don't want it around to be tempted by it - even asked them to hide it so you can't find it.

Now you might have a weakness for bread like I do. The way I get round that is I only buy enough for everybody else in the house and I don't buy any of the bread that I really, really like.

I'm not going to labour this point, after all your sensible enough to be doing this diet so I have to assume that your sensible enough to be able to work out how to keep the foods that you have a weakness for out of your own reach.

Shopping

The practicalities of any diet start in the store. It's in the store where you buy the things that you need to make sure that you eat the right foods.

More importantly it's where you do not buy the things you should not be eating so as not to have temptation constantly around you when you get back home.

If it's not in the cupboard or in the refrigerator - you can't be tempted by it.

That's why it's important that when you go shopping you have a list and particularly where food items are concerned you make sure you stick to it.

It really is that simple. I have provided weekly shopping list in the chapter 'Shopping Lists' in part two.

Get Support

Having this book will be an enormous help to you as

you go through your diet but nothing can really replace the encouragement of other people going through the same thing. That's why one of the things that we've set up is a website that acts as a meeting point for other people on the snack box diet.

There is a whole host of articles, videos and more on the website and you can join in on the forum absolutely free (you will need to sign up though)

Not only that, but if you can also find somebody who is trying to get fit and lose fat like you are, then getting together to help and support each other - even if it's only just once a week and maybe only by email - will be an enormous help to you both. And obviously, if you can gel with more than one other like-minded person who brings a positive influence to your gathering then that can only be another source of help and encouragement.

Sensible Fat Loss Rates.

By following this diet closely you should expect to lose up to three pounds or 1 1/2 kg of fat a week. This is both achievable and sustainable in the long run. Now you might be achieving a little more or a little less each week but what we're looking at - is the average weight loss over a number of weeks.

So that does mean on average someone following this diet would be able to lose roundabout thirty pounds or 15 kg over a 10 week period.

But remember, we're not primarily concerned with the actual weight that you lose. We are more concerned with the inches that you lose around the various parts of your body.

The reason for that is simple in that you should, as part of this diet, have started on some form of exercise which will be increasing the size of your muscles. Not only does exercise build muscle, when done he right way it also "burns" fat. So you will find you get results sooner.

And you could quite easily lose two pounds of fat in between measurements but, due to the exercise, have put back a pound of lean muscle.

If you were looking solely at how much weight you had lost, you might be disappointed thinking you'd only lost a pound of fat. Whereas the reality was far much better than that.

Remember too, that muscle fibre weighs a little bit more than the fat for the same volume.

Nearly Ready to Go

So by now you will have written down all the things that being overweight is stopping you from doing or achieving.

You've also made a note of all the things that you're missing out on because you're out of condition and overweight.

Even better, you will have written down a huge list of things that you will gain by becoming fitter, leaner and certainly healthier.

All these things are necessary in order for you to find out where you want to be, and how you want to be at the end of this journey to finding the new you.

You will have also cleared the house of anything that may tempt you as well.

10. MEASURING YOUR PROGRESS

In order to find out how to get to your fat loss goal, we need to find out where you are to start with.

You should have already described in writing the type of body that you want - (on list two) now it's time to find out exactly what your body is like now.

This does two things ...

By seeing the difference between how you want to be at the end of this diet and where you are now, you'll be able to see exactly the task that lies ahead of you. That way you'll have all the information you need so that there are no surprises later on.

By understanding the task i.e. how many inches/centimetres, pounds/kilograms need to be got rid of, you can more clearly determine the best way forward.

By the way, your actual weight now as much as the target weight you set yourself are actually not too much concern when using this diet. (I discuss why elsewhere) What we are more concerned with are your measurements as they provide a far more accurate appraisal of how well you're doing.

So without further ado let's get on with taking some measurements.

You are actually going to be taking quite a few measurements and in order for you not to get lost - I have prepared a chart for you to fill in. Try and do these as accurately as you can and always wear the same (or the same type of) clothing each time you take the measurements.

Take each measurement in centimetres or inches that's up to you. And enter them in the chart provided in part two.

You're only going to do this once a week so it's worth doing well!

It is worth noting that the measurements taken are not the same for men and women. That's mainly to take into account the differences in our physiology and of the way that both sexes put on fat in different ways and places. If you can, get a friend to help you take the measurements – it's just easier.

Mens Measurements

Around your neck Where a shirt collar would go.

Around your chest Just under your armpits more or less at nipple level.

Waist At the largest part.

Upper arm At the largest part of your upper arm, without flexing their muscles and your arms straight.

Forearm at the largest part of your forearm with your arms straight without flexing their muscles.

Thighs At the largest part of each leg measured separately.

Calves At the largest part of your calf.

Don't worry that you haven't as many measurements as the ladies. Men and women not only put on weight differently, they also lose it in other ways too. Now turn to the chapter 'Your

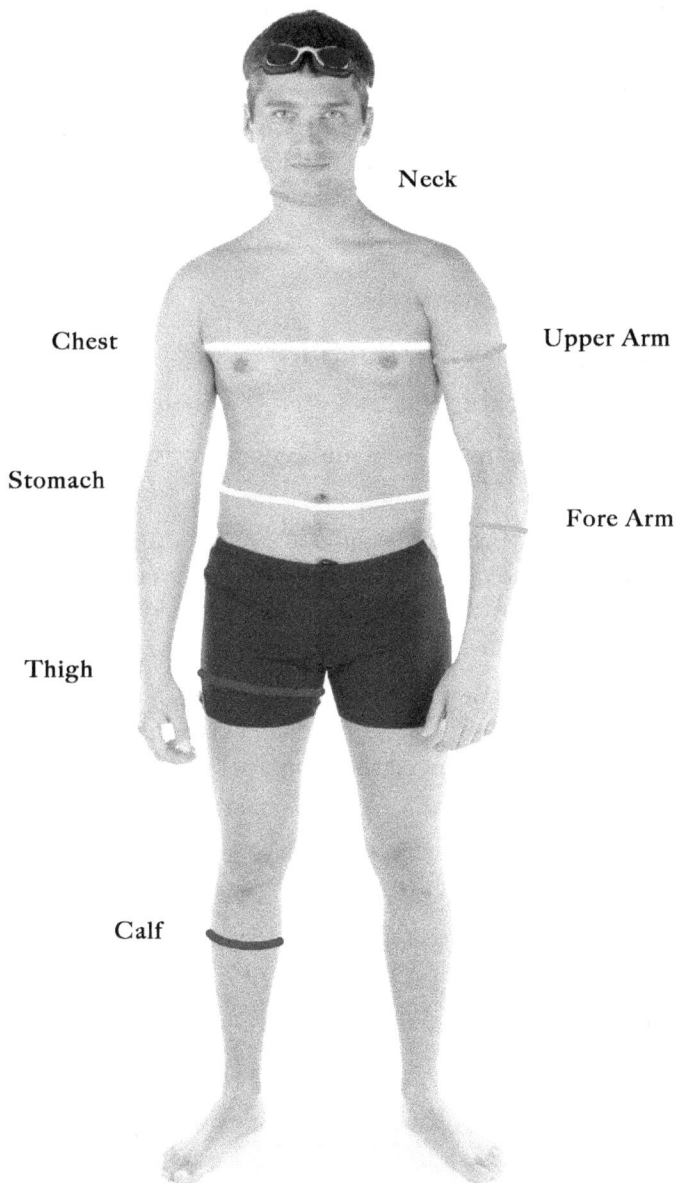

Neck

Chest

Upper Arm

Stomach

Fore Arm

Thigh

Calf

Progress Logs' and fill in the first column of the Mens table.

In the images of our sporty guy and girl you can see exactly where you need to measure and it really is worth the effort to do is as accurately. While most measurements are within easy reach for most people you may find it a bit easier to get a friend to help you if you find its a little difficult to do it right

Ladies Measurements

The measurements you need to take are...

Around your neck Where a shirt collar would go.

Around your chest As if you were getting measured for a bra...

1 - Keeping the measuring tape parallel with the ground, measure around your bra directly under your bust after expelling all air from your lungs - you want this measurement to be as small as possible.

2 - Standing straight, with your arms at your side, measure at the fullest part of your bust (while wearing a non-padded bra) making sure the measuring tape is parallel with the ground and not binding.

Upper arm At the largest part of your upper arm, without flexing your muscles and your arms straight.

Forearm At the largest part of your forearm with your arms straight without flexing their muscles.

Waist or Stomach At the largest part.

Hips At the level of the hip joint or the largest circumference of your hips.

Thighs At the largest part of each leg measured separately.

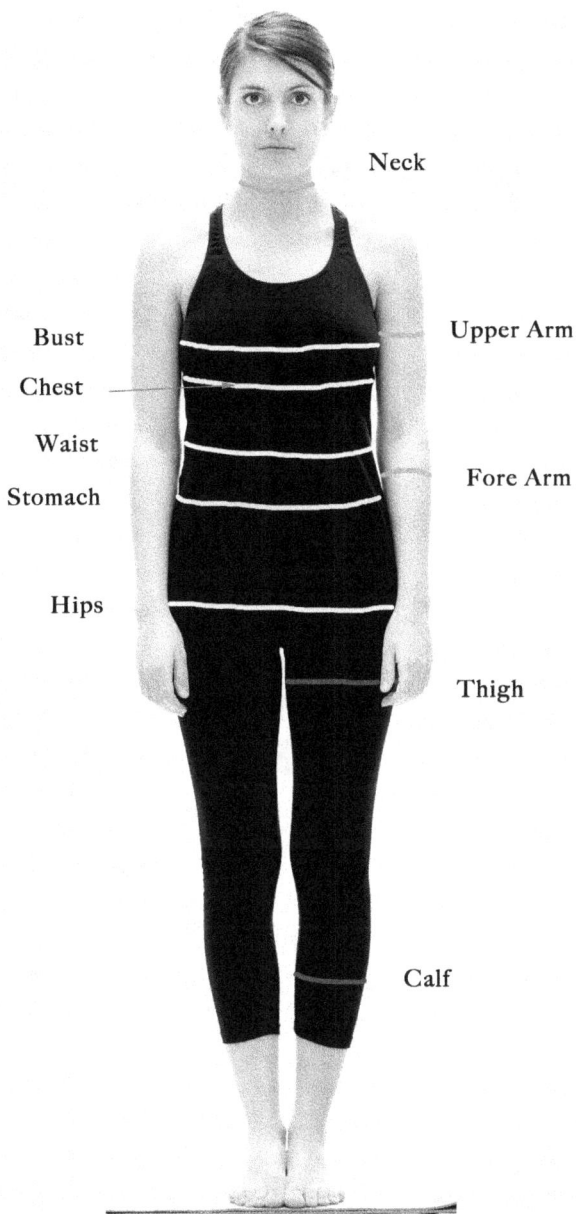

Neck

Upper Arm

Bust

Chest

Fore Arm

Waist

Stomach

Hips

Thigh

Calf

Calves At the largest part of your calf.

Now turn to the chapter 'Your Progress Logs' and fill in the first column of the Ladies table.

So, that's the measurements dealt with. Now, lets have a look at what's on the menu.

11. The Menus

The Daily Menu Planner

There are so many foods that you can eat each day that it could seem a bit bewildering when you first start this diet.

So in order to make it as easy as possible I prepare five weeks worth of lunch boxes just to get you started.

Obviously, once you get into the hang of things you'll be able to sort out exactly what you want to eat each day without any help from me.

The quantities given are enough for a fairly active person. But you will very quickly be able to gauge the quantities you require for yourself - probably within three or four days.

Frankly, if you find there's too much in the box then don't try and force yourself to eat it all. On the other hand, if you find you are running out of food by the end of the evening then there is nothing wrong with having more of the things included on the OK Foods list.

Don't forget though, these are just the background foods that you can eat - if you prefer - the daily staples.

As well as those, I have included over 30 different recipes that you can use throughout the five-week period. Some of the ingredients for these have been taken from the daily staples.

I've also included a shopping list for each week as well (In part two of the book). Obviously that makes life a lot easier.

When preparing the dishes, follow either the metric or imperial measurements! Don't mix them up as it could spoil that taste. And note that I assume the meats and fish you buy will be the ready to eat variety . Although if you prefer to cook these yourself - that's even better . You can batch cook a few days worth and keep them refrigerated

As there are so many dips and sauces available now days I'm certain you will have your favourites. You can eat them but just be sure to chose those that are low in sugar, fillers and carbohydrates and don't eat more than the amount recommended for each day - typically 25g a day.

Any ingredients shown in <u>underlined type</u> are NOT on the OK list but are included to add taste, variety and interest as well as top up vitamins a little. So for these few items - stick with the quantities given and never be tempted to over indulge your self on them.

Finally, your taste will be a little different to mine. Feel free to alter quantities slightly to suit your taste.

After all, Food is meant to be enjoyed.

12. MENU WEEK ONE

Monday

Dish of the Day - Tarragon and Honey Chicken

Tuesday

Dish of the Day - Grilled Chicken in a Tasty Orange Sauce

Wednesday

Dish of the Day – Parmesan on Fennel

Thursday

Dish of the Day – Broccoli and Bacon

Friday

Dish of the Day - Crab and Pea

Saturday

Dish of the Day - Turkey Apple and Walnut

Sunday

Dish of the Day - Tuna and Avocado

Monday's Dish of The Day
Tarragon and Honey Chicken

Ingredients for 1 Person

100g or 4oz or boneless skinless chicken breasts, five or six slices	1 lemon
	5 mL or 1 teaspoon of sesame oil
45 mL or 3 tablespoons of olive oil	5 mL or 1 teaspoon of clear honey
1 garlic clove, finely chopped	5g or 2 teaspoons of toasted sesame seeds
25g or half cup of watercress	
3 lettuce leaves	2 g or 1 teaspoon fresh tarragon, chopped
6 cherry tomatoes	

Preparations before you go...

Grate the rind and then juice the lemon. Pour 30 mL (2 tablespoons) of the olive oil into a small bowl and add 2 teaspoons of lemon rind and 5 mL (1 teaspoon) of the lemon juice, garlic, tarragon and a good pinch of salt and pepper. Rub this mixture over the sliced chicken and then cook in a hot griddle pan for 4 to 5 minutes until the meat is golden brown.

While that's cooking, combine the remaining olive oil, lemon juice, sesame oil, sesame seeds, honey, and add a sprinkle of salt and pepper.

Eating!

On a plate, make a bed of the lettuce and watercress. Arrange the chicken slices on top, artistically arranged the cherry tomatoes and then pour over the dressing. Decorate with watercress and enjoy.

Staples for Today:

Beef Roasted in Slices. 3 x 50g (2oz)

Chicken Breast 3 x 50g (2oz) in slices or strips

Smoked Salmon 75g (3oz) Slices

White Stilton x 50g (2oz)

Double Gloucester x 50g (2oz)

Goats Cheese x 50g (2oz)

Lettuce or 50g (2oz)

Tomatoes Sun Dried x 50g (2oz)

Chives x 25g (1oz) - Chopped fine and mixed with fish or other salad ingredients and a little dressing

Sauce or Dip of choice x 25g (1oz)

Almonds 50g (2oz)

Fromage Blanche x 50g (2oz)

Natural live yogurt 3 x 125g (5oz) pot

Apple x 1

Nutrition for Today:

Protein	191 g
Carbs	59 g
Fibre	9.7 g
Starch	0.2 g
Sugars	19.9 g
Fat	140 g
Water	565ml

Tuesday's Dish of The Day
Grilled Chicken in a Tasty Orange Sauce

Ingredients for 1

75g or 3oz of skinless boneless chicken breast halves

4 of 5 generous leaves of Romain lettuce - cleaned and chopped

6 Tangerine segments

25g or 1oz of grated carrot

15g or half an oz of fresh broccoli florets

15 mL or 1 table spoon of orange juice

15 mL or 1 table spoon of olive oil

15 mL or 1 table spoon of white wine vinegar

Preparation before you go ...

In a glass jar with a tight fitting lid, shake together the orange juice, olive oil, vinegar, honey, herb and garlic seasoning. Pour half of it into a bowl or cup.

Preheat the grill to a medium-high heat. Baste the chicken and cook for 6 to 8 minutes on each side boasting two or three times more during cooking.

Once the juices are running clear, removed from the grill and leave aside to cool then cut into strips.

Serving!

In your snack box bowl toss together the lettuce man doing segments broccoli and carrots. Place the grilled salad strips on top and drizzle over the remainder of the dressing and enjoy.

Staples for Today:

Chicken Breast 3 x 50g (2oz)
Smoked Salmon 75g (3oz)
  Slices
Bacon x 100g (4oz)
Crispy cooked broken up and
  put on salad with dressing
  of choice
Wensleydale x 50g (2oz)
Gloucester x 50g (2oz)
Quark x 50g (2oz)
Romain Lettuce x 100g (4oz)

Peppers Red x half
Carrots Grated 50g (2oz)
Sauce or Dip of choice x 25g
  (1oz)
Tangerine or Orange x1
Brazil nuts 50g (2oz)
Yogurt Greek x 1 pot - 125g
Natural live yogurt 3 x 125g
(5oz) pot

Nutrition for Today:

Protein	159 g
Carbs	57.6 g
Fibre	11 g
Starch	1.2 g
Sugars	35.5 g
Fat	159.9 g
Water	ml

Wednesday's Dish of The Day
Parmesan on Fennel Salad

Such a quick and easy one this and so tasty too.

Ingredients for 1

5 small fennel bulbs	chopped fresh dill
45 ml or 3 tablespoons of olive oil	5g or 1 tablespoon of chopped fresh flat leaf parsley
15 ml or 1 tablespoon of white wine vinegar	10 shavings of Parmesan cheese or quarter cup of grated Parmesan cheese
15ml or 1 tablespoon of	

Preparations before you go...

Grill or fry the bacon and allow it to cool. Cut the fennel bulbs lengthways, remove the core and then slice thinly.

Add the oil, vinegar, parsley, salt and pepper to a small glass jar and shake until the mixture is smooth and creamy.

Eating!

Throw the fennel into your bowl and add the most of the dressing and then toss well.

Lay the Parmesan over the top and pour over the remaining dressing. Eat either on it's own or as a side dish.

Staples for Today:

Smoked Salmon 75g (3oz) Slices – break up and mix with mushrooms and french dressing

Bacon x 100g (4oz) Crispy cooked broken up and put on the rest of salad with dressing of choice

Turkey Drumstick x 1 – With dressing or dip of choice

Swiss x 75g (3oz)

Gouda x 75g (3oz)

American Cheese x 50g (2oz)

Lettuce x 100g (4oz)

Mushrooms x 6 medium chopped or sliced fine

Fennel – Finochio - 5 small bulbs

<u>Beetroot cooked or pickled</u> x 50g (2oz) sliced or cubed

Sauce or Dip of choice x 25g (1oz)

Coconut Dried Sliced x 50g (2oz)

Fromage Blanche x 50g (2oz)

Natural live yogurt 3 x 125g (5oz) pot

Tip:

You have bacon a few times this week - why not cook it all at once.

Nutrition for Today:

Protein	146.8 g
Carbs	59.9 g
Fibre	8.9 g
Starch	0.2 g
Sugars	18 g
Fat	152.6 g
Water	457 ml

Thursday's Dish of The Day
Broccoli and Bacon

Such a simple dish this one and just the ticket if you like crunchy raw veggie's. If you want to add other veggies from the OK list then feel free to do so – as you wish.

Ingredients for 1

25g or 1oz of fresh broccoli florets.

25g or 1oz of bacon cooked and crumbled.

15g or half an oz of raisins.

25g or 1oz of sunflower seeds (shelled).

30 mL or 1 tablespoon of mayonnaise.

1 teaspoon of honey.

1 teaspoon of vinegar.

Preparations before you go...

Grill or fry the bacon and allow to cool. In a small bowl combine the broccoli, bacon, sunflower seeds and raisins. In a sealable jar - mix together the mayonnaise honey and vinegar.

Eating!

About one hour before eating pour the sauce over the salad and toss to coat well. Nicer chilled before eating. It can't get any simpler than that!

Staples for Today:

Bacon x 100g (4oz)
Crispy cooked broken up and
   put on salad with dressing
   of choice or see above.
Turkey Drumstick x 1
Crab Meat - 1 small tin or 50g
(2oz) -
 Cooked fresh or tinned
   broken up and mixed with
   salad, olives and a sprinkle
   of cashews

Shropshire Blue x 50g (2oz)
Leerdammer x 50g (2oz)
Munster x 50g (2oz)
Lettuce Iceberg x 100g (4oz)
Cucumber x 50g (2oz)
Olives Black x 20
Sauce or Dip of choice x 25g
   (1oz)
Cashews 50g (2oz)
Natural live yogurt 2 x 125g
(5oz) pot

Nutrition for Today:

Protein	150.4 g
Carbs	67.9 g
Fibre	9.5 g
Starch	1 g
Sugars	10 g
Fat	173 g
Water	510 ml

Friday's Dish of The Day
Crab and Pea Salad

Seafood and peas are a tradition in many parts of the world – it seems they were made for each other and the same goes here, but add in the bacon - and it takes on flavour altogether much tastier than it sounds.

Ingredients for 1

75g or 3oz of peas, fresh or frozen (thawed out obviously)

50g or 2oz of crab meat

2 strips of bacon cooked and crumbled

30 mL or 2 tablespoonfuls of mayonnaise

25g or 1oz of onion finely chopped

Salt and pepper to taste

Preparation before you go...

In a small bowl, combine the peas, crab, bacon, onion and mayonnaise. Cover tightly and keep cold until serving.

Eating!

Add a little more mayo if needed. Just don't pig out!

Staples for Today:

Turkey Drumstick x 2 With
   dressing or dip of choice
Crab Meat - 1 small tin or 50g
   (2oz) -
Cooked fresh or tinned
   broken up and mixed with
   salad and cubed mimolette
   cheese
Ham Slices - 3 x 50g (2oz) –
   Filled with Soft cheese of
   choice and rolled
Romano x 50g (2oz)
Mimolette x 75g (3oz)

Reblochon x 50g (2oz)
Lettuce x 100g (4oz)
Romaine x 100g (4oz)
Tomatoes x 2 medium
Dill Pickle - Small x 4
Sauce or Dip of choice x 25g
   (1oz)
Coconut Fresh 50g (2oz)
Apricot Fresh x1
 Fromage Blanche x 50g (2oz)
Natural live yogurt x 2 125g
   pots

Nutrition for Today:

Protein	169 g
Carbs	62.8 g
Fibre	16 g
Starch	0.7 g
Sugars	36.3 g
Fat	119 g
Water	1208 ml

Saturday's Dish of The Day
Turkey Apple and Walnut Salad

Succulent turkey, sweet apples and a touch of nuttiness from the walnuts all go together to give a sublime combination of tastes and textures that your taste buds won't be able to resist.

Ingredients for 1

1 turkey breast, grilled or fried and sliced into strips

1 small dessert apple, cord and chopped roughly

25g or 1oz of shelled walnuts, roughly chopped

25g or 1oz of white cabbage, finely shredded

1 celery stick, thinly sliced

3 large radishes. Cut the roots and tops off and slice thinly.

15g or half an oz of stoned raisins

30 mL or two tablespoons of soured cream

1 teaspoon of lemon juice

Salt and black pepper to taste

Preparation before you go ...

Pour the apple chunks into a bowl and sprinkle with lemon juice (so they don't go brown) add in two thirds of the chopped walnuts, cabbage, celery, radishes and raisins. Cover and keep cool.

Eating!

Uncover your bowl and add most of the soured cream and mix well. Place the turkey strips on top, pour over the rest of the cream, sprinkle a little salt and pepper and top off with the rest of the walnuts.

Staples for Today:

Crab Meat - 1 small tin or 50g (2oz) - Cooked fresh or tinned broken up and mixed with Mustard and Cress french dressing and topped with Hazelnuts

Ham Slices - 3 x 50g (2oz)

Turkey Breast x1 - RTE

Monterey Jack x 50g (2oz) Dry x 50g (2oz)

Port Salut x 50g (2oz)

Petit-Suisse x 50g (2oz)

Mustard and Cress or 50g (2oz)

Pepper Green x half

Onions x 50g (2oz) - white or red as you prefer

Carrots 50g (2oz) - Straws or grated and mixed with a little french dressing

Sauce or Dip of choice x 25g (1 oz)

1 small Apple

Wallnuts 50g (2oz)

Yogurt Greek x 1 pot – 125gr

Natural live yogurt x 2 125g pots

Nutrition for Today:

Protein	109 g
Carbs	75.4 g
Fibre	16 g
Starch	1.2 g
Sugars	34.1 g
Fat	87.5 g
Water	724.8 ml

Sunday's Dish of The Day
Tuna and Avocado Salad

The slightly salty flavour of the tuna goes well with the avocado – but really, it's the dressing that ties it all together.

Ingredients for 1

100g or 4oz of tuna in brine
Half a small avocado stoned, peeled and cubed
Half a celery stick, roughly chopped
1 radish, finely sliced
10 mL or 2 teaspoons of
lemon juice
10 mL or 2 teaspoons of tarragon vinegar
1 spring onion, finely chopped
Pinch of cayenne pepper
salt and pepper to taste

Dressing

30 mL or two tablespoons of tarragon vinegar
15 mL or one tablespoon of olive oil
45 mL or three tablespoons of peanut oil
3 mL or half a teaspoon of Dijon mustard
3 mL or half a teaspoon of lemon juice
15 mg or half an oz of fresh dill, chopped

Preparations before you go ...

Place all ingredients for the dressing in a glass jar with a tight fitting lid and shake until creamy.

Eating!

Toss all the ingredients for the main dish together in a bowl. Place the fish on top and pour over as much of the dressing as you like. Add any other salad stuff you like. Fill the other half of the avocado with mayo and sprinkle over a generous pinch of cayenne pepper.

Staples for Today:

Ham Slices - 3 x 50g (2oz) -
  Filled with soft cheese of
  choice and rolled (Finely
  chop a few radishes and add
  to cheese - if you like them)
Turkey Breast x1 - Sliced as
  you like it. Goes great with
  the cranberries
Tuna in brine - 1 small tin -
  Eat as you want or mix with
  salad
Leicester x 75g (3oz)

Monterey Jack x 50g (2oz)
Petit Suisse x 75g (3oz)
Celery- 2 sticks
Tomatoes x 2 medium
Radishes x 9
Sauce or Dip of choice x 25g
  (1 oz)
Macadamia 50g (2oz)
Cranberies 25g (1oz)
Fromage Blanche x 50g (2oz)
Natural live yogurt x 2 125g
  pots

Nutrition for Today:

Protein	127 g
Carbs	55.3 g
Fibre	13.5 g
Starch	0.8 g
Sugars	32.6 g
Fat	126.2 g
Water	919 ml

Nutrition for Week One – Recap...

If you have eaten everything in the menus and on the staples lists for week one - then you will have had a daily average of the following ...

Protein	150.7g
Carbs	62.6g
Fiber	12.1g
Fat	136.9g
Saturated	52.3g
Omega-3	2.1g
Omega-6	12.6 g
Cholesterol	400.8mg

So Well done! You have sailed through your first week on the Snack Box Diet.

Don't forget to go and measure yourself to see how you have progressed.

13. Menu Week Two

Monday

Dish of the Day - Fresh Tomato Salad

Tuesday

Dish of the Day - Salami, Tomatoes and Mozzarella

Wednesday

Dish of the Day – Roast Beef and Palm Hearts

Thursday

Dish of the Day – Thousand Islands Chicken

Friday

Dish of the Day - Duck Waldorf

Saturday

Dish of the Day - Smoked Haddock with Egg and Beans

Sunday

Dish of the Day - Pork and Spinach Salad

Monday's Dish of The Day
Fresh Tomato Salad

This is a simple but lovely dish eaten on its own. As a bonus it is also delicious with any cold meat and cheese too. So you can do as you like with this one.

Ingredients for 1

2 tomatoes

45 ml or 3 tablespoons of olive oil

15 ml or 1 tablespoon of white

5 ml or 1 teaspoon of honey

wine vinegar

5 ml or 1 teaspoon full of chopped chives or tarragon

Salt and pepper to taste

Preparation before you go ...

Thinly slice the tomatoes and arrange them in a shallow dish. Mix the oil honey and vinegar together and sprinkle over the tomatoes. Sprinkle over the chopped tarragon or chives, cover and leave to chill for at least an hour in the refrigerator, turning the mixture over once or twice.

Eating!

Uncover, season with salt and pepper and enjoy with the rest of todays offering.

Staples for Today:

Turkey Breast x1 –Broken and mixed with salad

Tuna in brine – 100g (4oz) small tin - Eat as you want or mix with salad

Pork/Danish Salami - 100g (4oz)- Put your favourite cream cheese and dill pickles cut in straws in the middle and roll up like a sausage

Lancashire x 50g (2oz)

Airedale x 50g (2oz)

Jubilee Blue x 50g (2oz)

Roquette 100g (4oz)

Celery x 2 sticks Whole or chopped in to 1cm slices if you prefer

Spring Onions - 50g (2oz) Sauce or Dip of choice x 25g (1 oz)

Hummus 50g

Peanuts 50g (2oz)

Fromage Blanche x 100g (4oz)

Natural live yogurt x 1 pot 125g (5oz)

Nutrition for Today:

Protein	122.2 g
Carbs	59.2 g
Fibre	14.8 g
Starch	0.4 g
Sugars	30.6 g
Fat	199.2 g
Water	710 ml

Tuesday's Dish of The Day
Salami, Tomatoes and Mozzarella

A simple dish to make and totally delicious. Works with any type of salami too.

Ingredients for 1

50g or 2oz of salami
1 tomato, diced
3 fresh basil leaves chopped
25g or 1oz of mozzarella,
   sliced

10 mL or 2 teaspoons of olive
   oil
5 mL or 1 teaspoon of
   balsamic or wine vinegar
Salt and pepper

Preparation before you go ...

None... really

Eating!

Divide the salami slices into quarters and throw into your bowl. Add the tomatoes, mozzarella, basil and season with a little salt and pepper. Drizzle over the olive oil and vinegar and toss well.

Staples for Today:

Tuna in Oil - 1 small tin
Pork/Danish Salami - 100g
 (4oz)
Chicken Sliced 3 x 50g (2oz)
Jarlsberg x 75g (3oz)
Beaufort x 75g (3oz)
Curd x 50g (2oz)
Sorrel 100g (4oz)
Tomatoes x 2 medium
Chives - 20g - Chopped fine
and mixed with fish or other
 salad
Sauce or Dip of choice x 25g
 (1 oz)
Pecans 50g (2oz)
Blueberries Fresh x 50g (2oz)
 Fromage Blanche x 50g
 (2oz)
Natural live yogurt x 1 pot
 125gr

Nutrition for Today:

Protein	142 g
Carbs	45.7 g
Fibre	10.3 g
Starch	0.4 g
Sugars	25.2 g
Fat	162.3 g
Water	712 ml

71

Wednesday's Dish of The Day
Roast Beef and Palm Hearts

This is a very tasty dish (which is ideal for using up leftover roast) While it can be eaten on its own, it's also very nice with a fresh green salad. You can use any roasted meat or poultry in place of the beef if you prefer. It does taste better when the meat is on the rare side.

Ingredients for 1

100g or 4oz of roast beef (rare)

2 Palm hearts, sliced finely

1 hard-boiled egg, roughly chopped

15 mL or 1 table spoon of olive oil

5 mL or 1 teaspoon of wine vinegar

3 mL or 1/2 teaspoon Dijon mustard

1 anchovy fillet, finely chopped

Half teaspoon finely chopped capers

1 level teaspoon chopped chives

1 level teaspoon of chopped parsley

Preparation before you go ...

For the sauce, mix the oil, vinegar and mustard thoroughly and then add the capers, anchovy fillets, chives, parsley and a little pepper.

Slice the beef into matchstick sized strips then pour over the sauce. Cover and leave the meat to marinate for at least an hour.

Eating!

Arrange the palm heart slices around the edge of your plate and pile the meat in the centre and garnish with the chopped hard-boiled egg.

Staples for Today:

Pork/Danish Salami - 100g (4oz)- Put Your favourite cream cheese and chopped olive in the middle and roll up like a sausage

Beef roasted and sliced 3 x 50g (2oz)

Sardines in Tomato - Small tin - Great on salad as a separate dish

Gruyère x 50g (2oz)

Canadian Cheddar x 75g (3oz)

Gorgonzola x 50g (2oz)

Watercress 100g (4oz)

Peppers Red x half

Olives Green x 20

Sauce or Dip of choice x 25g (1 oz)

Pine-nuts 50g (2oz)

Yogurt Greek 125g

Nutrition for Today:

Protein	157.9 g
Carbs	41.7 g
Fibre	6.7 g
Starch	0.7 g
Sugars	21.5 g
Fat	213 g
Water	539 ml

Thursday's Dish of The Day
Thousand Islands Chicken

A slightly exotic mix but very tasty. Also works very well with turkey or other poultry.

Ingredients for 1

25g or 1 oz of cooked chicken, diced

1 palm heart, diced

25g or 1 oz of cucumber, peeled and diced

1 small spring onion, sliced thinly

Half a stick of celery, chopped into 1 cm pieces

30 mL or 2 tablespoons of French dressing. (Any one from this book or ready made)

1 small garlic clove, crushed

2 or 3 lettuce leaves, torn into bite-size pieces

1 hard-boiled egg, quartered

15 mL or one table spoon of mayonnaise

15 mL or one tablespoon tomato ketchup

Generous pinch of paprika

Preparation before you go...

Put the palm hearts, chicken, cucumber, celery and onions in a bowl. Mix the paprika into the French dressing and then pour it on and mix well. Cover and leave to cool.

Eating!

Cover the plate with the lettuce and pile the chicken salad in the centre and arrange the egg slices around the chicken.

Mix together the mayonnaise and tomato ketchup and then spoon over the egg slices.

Staples for Today:

Chicken cooked, diced or sliced 3 x 50g (2oz) or diced.
Sardines in Tomato - Small tin
Pepperoni Sausage 100g (4oz)-
Grafton Village Cheddar x 75g (3oz)
Cantal x 75g (3oz)
Dauphin x 50g (2oz)
Endives - 100g (4oz)
Mushrooms - 6 medium

chopped or sliced fine
Cucumber x 50g (2oz)
Sauce or Dip of choice x 25g (1 oz)
Pistachios 50g (2oz)
Figs Fresh x1
Fromage Blanche x 50g (2oz)
Natural live yogurt x 1 pot 125gr

Nutrition for Today:

Protein	155.8 g
Carbs	60.2 g
Fibre	14.3 g
Starch	1.7 g
Sugars	31.3 g
Fat	178.2 g
Water	888 ml

Friday's Dish of the Day
Duck Waldorf

I love this dish. It's simple and easy to prepare and makes a real treat on any day of the week.

Ingredients for 1

75g or 3oz of duck breast, roasted ready to eat, roughly sliced

1 <u>small red apple</u>, cord and cubed

10 mL or 2 teaspoons of lemon juice

2 g or half a teaspoon of caster sugar

30 mL or 2 tablespoons of mayonnaise

half a stick of celery, roughly chopped

15g or half an oz of shelled walnuts

3 or 4 lettuce leaves

Preparations before you go ...

Mix together the lemon juice, caster sugar and one tablespoon of mayonnaise. Add in the apple cubes and stir to make sure they are thoroughly covered in the dressing. Leave to stand for 30 minutes.

Add the walnuts, celery and one more spoon of mayonnaise to the mix and stir thoroughly. Cover and refrigerate.

Eating!

Place the lettuce leaves on the plate, pile the mix in the centre and arrange the duck over the top. Add a bit more mayonnaise if you need it.

Staples for Today:

Sardines in Tomato - Small tin
- Great with olives and salad
or as a separate dish
Pepperoni Sausage 100g
(4oz)-
Duck Breast -150grs (6oz)-
Loverly on its own sliced
with and smeared with a
little fig jam or marmalade
Emmental x 50g (2oz)

Cheddar x 75g (3oz)
Fresh Mozzarella x 75g (3oz)
Escarole x 100g (4oz)
Cucumber x 50g (2oz)
Olives Black x 20
Sauce or Dip of choice x 25g
(1 oz)
Pumpkin seeds 50g (2oz)
Natural live yogurt x 2 pots of
125gr

Nutrition for Today:

Protein	161.3 g
Carbs	62.6 g
Fibre	14.4 g
Starch	1.8 g
Sugars	37.3 g
Fat	181.6 g
Water	984 ml

Saturday's Dish of the Day
Smoked Haddock with Egg and Beans

This dish actually works quite nicely when the egg and beans are still warm. In fact, if you are doing this at home try using a poached egg instead of boiled.

Ingredients for 1

150g or 6oz of smoked haddock

100g or 4oz of trimmed French beans

1 egg, hard-boiled, quartered

45 mL or three tablespoons of olive oil

15 mL or 1 table spoon of cider vinegar

5 mL or 1 teaspoon of whole grain mustard

25g or 1 oz lettuce or greens of your choice

Preparations before you go ...

Boil the beans for 3 to 5 minutes until cooked but still with that little bit of crunch. Drain and cool.

Whisk the mustard, and vinegar, and oil together add a little salt and pepper to taste then pour most of it over the cooled beans.

Eating!

Place the salad leaves into your bowl and break the haddock over it, add in the beans and half the dressing and toss thoroughly. Arrange the eggs over the top and drizzle over the rest of the dressing.

Staples for Today:

Pepperoni Sausage 100g (4oz)- Chopped or sliced in with the fish or mixed with the salad

Duck Breast -150grs -

Haddock Smoked - 150g (6oz) Break up and mix with chopped dills and a dollop of mayo

Dutch Mimolette x 75g (3oz)

Cheshire x 50g (2oz)

Monastery Cheeses x 50g (2oz)

Alfalfa sprouts 50g (2oz)

Tomatoes x 2 medium

Dill Pickle x 3

Sauce or Dip of choice x 25g (1 oz)

Sesame seeds 50g (2oz)

Gooseberries Fresh x half cup

Fromage Blanche x 50g (2oz)

Nutrition for Today:

Protein	164.6 g
Carbs	59.9 g
Fibre	20.6 g
Starch	g
Sugars	13.9 g
Fat	176.9 g
Water	980 ml

Sunday's Dish of the Day
Pork and Spinach Salad

A great dish for the weekend and you can use lamb or pork – whichever you prefer. And it works well with leftovers too. It's really nice to eat just cooked, but if you want to eat it 'SnackBox Style' then do let the meat and vegetables cool before you put them in your snack box and then refrigerate until your ready.

Ingredients for 1

100g or 4oz of black eyed peas pre-cooked rinsed and drained

75g of fresh spinach (stems removed)

50g or 2oz of pork tenderloin cut into strips

15g or half an oz of fresh mushrooms

Half a celery stick sliced in 1 cm pieces

15g or half an oz of pimentos drained

6 olives - stoned and cut in half

1 garlic clove finally minced

1 or 2 tablespoons of Italian salad dressing (See page 134)

Preparation...

Place your spinach leaves in the bottom of your snack box bowl.

In another bowl, combine the vegetable - peas, mushrooms, celery, pimentos, olives and green onions then pour over the salad dressing and mix thoroughly.

In a medium-sized skillet or frying pan, sauté the garlic in the olive oil for 30 seconds, add the pork strips and stir fry for 2 to 3 minutes. Add the vegetable mixture and stir once or twice to mix thoroughly and then take off the heat.

Pour the meat and vegetable mixture over the spinach leaves

Staples for Today:

and eat it straight away.

Duck Breast -150g (6oz) –
Sliced finely

Haddock Smoked - 150g
(6oz)

Pork or Lamb Roasted in
Slices - 150g (6oz)

Double Worcester x 50g (2oz)

Devon Blue x 50g (2oz)

Fontainebleau x 50g (2oz)

Dandelion leaves x 100g (4oz)

Pepper Green x half sliced
finely

Onions x 50g (2oz) - White or
red as you prefer

Sauce or Dip of choice x 25g
(1 oz)

Sunflower seeds 50g (2oz)

Yogurt Greek 125g or 5oz

Fontainebleau cheese is very creamy and it goes well with fruit a little chopped dried fruit and some crushed nuts. Or you have any cream cheese in it's place.

Nutrition for Today:

Protein	148.8 g
Carbs	58.8 g
Fibre	17.9 g
Starch	0.2 g
Sugars	13.1 g
Fat	103.9 g
Water	741 ml

Nutrition for Week Two — Recap...

If you have eaten everything in the menus and on the staples lists for the second week of becoming the new you - then you will have had a daily average of the following ...

Protein	150g
Carbs	55 g
Fiber	14.1 g
Fat	173.6 g
Saturated	58.4 g
Omega-3	2.9 g
Omega-6	19.3 g
Cholesterol	534.6 mg

So Well done yet again! You have powered through your second week on the Snack Box Diet.

Don't forget to go and measure yourself again to see how you have progressed.

14. MENU WEEK THREE

Monday

Dish of the Day - Zingy Walnut, Roquefort and Endives Salad

Tuesday

Dish of the Day - Lamb and Mint with Avocado

Wednesday

Dish of the Day – Prawns and Mushroom

Thursday

Dish of the Day – Prosciutto and Spinach Salad

Friday

Dish of the Day - Smoked Salmon Salad

Saturday

Dish of the Day - Beef, Cucumber and Soured Cream

Sunday

Dish of the Day - Berry Nice Chicken Salad

Monday's Dish of the Day
Zingy Walnut, Roquefort and Endives Salad

Another great combination of tastes and textures that somehow bring the taste buds alive and demanding more. - So, indulge them a little. It's a simple dish and quite light and it works well as a side dish too.

Ingredients for 1

One plump head of endives
25g or 1 oz of chopped
   walnuts
25g or 1 oz of crumbled
   Roquefort
30ml or 2 tablespoons of olive
   oil

5 ml or 1 teaspoon fresh
   lemon juice
5 ml or 1 teaspoon of grated
   orange zest
5 ml or 1 teaspoon fresh
   orange juice

Preparation before you go...

Separate the leaves of endives, wash well and dry

In a bowl (or glass jar) mix together the oil, lemon and orange juice, orange zest, crumbled Roquefort cheese and add salt and pepper to taste.

Eating!

Arrange your endive leaves on your plate.

Just before serving, pour the dressing over the endives and sprinkle with the walnuts.

Staples for Today:

Haddock Smoked - 75g (3oz)
Lamb Roasted in Cubes - 150g
   (6oz)- Cubes and mixed
   with mayonnaise, a little
   curry powder and eaten
   with salad
Turkey Leg - Just eat it off the
   bone.
Dorset Blue x 50g (2oz)
Roquefort x 50g (2oz)
Paneer Cheese x 50g (2oz)

Endives x 100g (4oz)
Tomatoes Cherry x 10 or 12
Radishes x 9 or 10
Sauce or Dip of choice x 25g
   (1 oz)
Walnuts 50g (2oz)
Orange x 1 small one
   Fromage Blanche 125 g (5oz)

Queso Blanco, Queso fresco, cottage or Farmers cheese make a good alternative to paneer cheese.

Nutrition for Today:

Protein	230.6 g
Carbs	34.7 g
Fibre	10.5 g
Starch	0.4 g
Sugars	17.9 g
Fat	203.3 g
Water	859 ml

Tuesday's Dish of the Day
Lamb and Mint with Avocado

Eating mint with lamb is a delicious age-old tradition particularly with the Anglo-Saxons. Adding avocado to the mix is simply inspired.

Ingredients for 1

75g or 3oz of roasted lamb, cut into strips

1 ripe avocado

1 small lime

100 mL or 7 tablespoons of soured cream

2 sprigs of fresh mint

Ground black pepper and salt

Preparation before you go ...

Slice a wedge out of the lime and set aside. Squeeze 10 mL or 2 teaspoons of out of the rest of the lime and set aside. Finely chopped one sprig of mint.

Halve the avocado, take out the stone and spoon out the flesh into a bowl. Sprinkle over the lime juice and mash with a fork. Mix in the soured cream and chopped mint and season with a little salt-and-pepper to taste. Cover tightly and chill for at least two hours.

Eating!

Arrange the strips of lamb on the plate, spoon over the avocado mixture and garnish with the other sprig of fresh mint and lime wedge. – Give an extra squeeze of lime if you want to.

More mint can be added if you like the minty taste

Staples for Today:

Lamb Slices - 150g (6oz)– Eat with the chopped beetroot mixed with salad and a light french dressing

Turkey Leg - Just eat in of the bone.

Cod Dried - 50g (2oz) – Also lovely with beet root and french dressing

Derby x 75g (3oz)

Saint-Paulin x 75g (3oz)

Feta x 75g (3oz)

Iceberg x100g (4oz)

Spring Onions - 50g (2oz)

Beetroot x 50g (2oz) sliced or cubed

Tomatoes x 2 medium

Celery x 2 sticks chopped in to 1cm slices if you prefer

Sauce or Dip of choice x 20g

Almonds 50g (2oz)

Natural live yogurt x 1 pot 125gr

There are several varieties of Saint Paulin cheese. One is a semi hard cheese made from sheeps milk and is very tasty. Another creamy and mild similar to Avarti. You can substitute which ever cheese you prefer for this one

Nutrition for Today:

Protein	269 g
Carbs	59.2 g
Fibre	21 g
Starch	0.5 g
Sugars	30.6 g
Fat	211 g
Water	1190 ml

Wednesday's Dish of the Day
Prawns and Mushroom

A superbly refreshing cold dish which goes well on its own.

Ingredients for 1

50g or 2oz of large mushrooms, peeled and thinly sliced

25g or 1 oz of shelled prawns

30 mL or two tablespoons of olive oil

10 mL of 2 teaspoons of lemon juice

1 clove of garlic, crushed

5 mg or a quarter of an oz of parsley

Salt and pepper to taste

Preparations before you go ...

Slice the mushrooms thinly and arrange them in a shallow dish.

Mix the oil, lemon juice, garlic and pepper together and pour over the mushrooms. Turn the slices of mushrooms over so they're evenly covered.

Cover and leave this mixture in the refrigerator for about an hour before serving turning a few times if you can..

Eating!

Uncover the mushrooms, add a little more olive oil if necessary and turn to cover evenly. Arrange the prawns around the mushrooms and sprinkle over a little salt to your taste. Garnish with parsley.

Staples for Today:

Shelled Prawns - 50g (2oz) –
   The ready to eat ones
Lamb Roasted in slices - 150gr
Beef roasted sliced 150g (6oz)
Derby x 50g (2oz)
Cheddar x 75g (3oz)
Boursin x 55g (2oz)
Iceberg x100g (4oz)
Celery x 2 sticks chopped in
   to 1cm slices if you prefer

Spring Onions - 50g (2oz)
Tomatoes Sun Dried x 30g
   (2oz) sliced or cubed
Sauce or Dip of choice x 20g
Almonds 50g (2oz)
Fromage Blanche 125g or
   (5oz)

   Prawns = Shrimps - A jar or tin of the precooked variety
are easiest to use.

Nutrition for Today:

Protein	141 g
Carbs	60 g
Fibre	14.1 g
Starch	0.8 g
Sugars	23.3 g
Fat	223.4 g
Water	562 ml

Thursday's Dish of the Day
Prosciutto and Spinach Salad

This is a totally refreshing dish that can have as much bite as you like simply by adding a little more or less oil to the dressing. You can use any dry smoked meat with this recipe.

Ingredients for 1

25g or 1 oz of prosciutto

25g or 1 oz of goats cheese, crumbled

25g or 1 oz of washed baby spinach

5 mL or 1 teaspoon of olive oil

15 mL or 1 tablespoon balsamic vinegar

5 mL or 1 teaspoon dark sesame oil (optional but worth it)

Salt and pepper to taste

Preparations before you go ...

Put the olive oil, sesame oil and vinegar into a glass jar with a tight fitting lid and shake together.

Eating!

Put the spinach leaves in a bowl, pour over the dressing and toss well.

Arrange the prosciutto on your plate, place the spinach on top of that and top off with the goats cheese.

Staples for Today:

Cod Dried - 50g (2oz)
Prosciutto - 100g (4oz)Mix with salad of the day and either cover with dressing or eat with Sauce or Dip of choice
Chicken Drumstick x 2 Best eaten straight off the bone
Cairnsmore x 75g (3oz)

Tomme cheese x 75g (3oz)
Goats cheese dry x 50g (2oz)
Mustard and Cress 50g (2oz)
Peppers Red x half
Olives Green x 20
Sauce or Dip of choice x 20g
Cashews 50g (2oz)
Yogurt Greek 125 g (6oz)

Cairnsmore cheese is made from sheeps milk and comes in several varieties - substitutes any cheese you prefer if you can't find it locally.

Nutrition for Today:

Protein	200 g
Carbs	40.7 g
Fibre	6.5 g
Starch	0 g
Sugars	7.9 g
Fat	106 g
Water	460 ml

Friday's Dish of the Day
Smoked Salmon Salad

This is a simple and quick dish to prepare and in fact needs no preparation at home as it can all be made just before you want to eat it.

Ingredients for 1

100g all 4oz of ready to eat mixed salad leaves

150g or 6oz of smoked salmon, sliced

15g or half oz of chopped walnut pieces

5 mL or 1 teaspoon of olive oil

6 Cherry tomatoes

Lemon wedge or 1 teaspoon of lemon juice

Salt and pepper to taste

Preparation before you go ...

None really - it can all be done as you want to eat it

Eating!

Simply place the salad leaves on the plate, lay the salmon strips over the top and top off with the walnuts. Throw on the cherry tomatoes and then sprinkle over the oil and lemon juice. Season to taste with salt and pepper.

Staples for Today:

Prosciutto - 100g (4oz)
Chicken Drumstick x 2 Best
   eaten straight off the bone
Smoked Salmon x 1 small
   pack
Caerphilly x 75g (3oz)
Yorkshire Blue x 50g (2oz)
Goats cheese x 75g (3oz)
Tomatoes Cherry x 10 or 12
Mushrooms - 6 medium

chopped or sliced fine
Mixed salad greens 200g or
   (8oz) Pack
Carrots Grated 50g (2oz)
Sauce or Dip of choice x 20g
Coconut Dried Sliced 50g
   (2oz)
Plums Fresh Small x1
 Fromage Blanche x 50g (2oz)

Nutrition for Today:

Protein	131 g
Carbs	54.4 g
Fibre	14.3 g
Starch	1.2 g
Sugars	27.3 g
Fat	138.2 g
Water	1000 ml

Saturday's Dish of the Day
Beef, Cucumber and Soured Cream

This is a great recipe to use when you want to finish up meat left over from a roast. It takes a little bit of preparation so it's probably best left to the weekend. Also, there's nothing stopping you from making it in advance to take with you in your snack box.

Frankly this is too good to eat on your own so I've given you the quantities for two people - just this once.

Ingredients for 2

4 Beef slices x 50g or 2oz each
1 small cucumber, peeled and cubed (1 cm)
15g or 1 tablespoon plain flour
15 mL or 1 table spoon of white wine vinegar
1 egg yolk
30 mL or 2 tablespoons of olive oil

75 mL or 5 tablespoons of soured cream
1 tablespoon of finely chopped chives
Quarter of a teaspoon of salt
Quarter of a teaspoon caster sugar
Quarter of a teaspoon of Dijon mustard

Preparations before you go ...

Add the flour, salt and mustard to a heavy-based pan with 10 mL or two teaspoonfuls of water. Blend well over a low heat then gradually add the vinegar and 15 mL or one tablespoon of water and continue cooking until the mixture has thickened to a smooth sauce.

Take the pan off the heat and allow to cool for a minute then beat in the egg yolk then beat in the oil and the few drops at the time. Pour into a suitable bowl, cover and refrigerate for about an hour.

Eating!

Stir in the soured cream and cucumber just before eating. Fold or roll the beef into tubes place on your plate and spoon over generous helpings of the cucumber sauce over the top and around the sides.

Staples for Today:

Chicken Drumstick x 2 Best eaten straight offf the bone
Salmon Tinned in brine x 1 small tin – Dowse with lemon or lime juice and eat with salad
Beef Slices 3 x 50g (2oz) each
White Stilton x 50g (2oz)
Airedale x 50g (2oz)

Coeur de Chevre x 75g (3oz)
Roquette-Arugula 50g (2oz)
Cucumber x 50g (2oz)
Olives Black x 20
Sauce or Dip of choice x 20g
Coconut Fresh 50g (2oz)
Natural live yogurt x 1 pot 125gr50

Nutrition for Today:

Protein	174 g
Carbs	26.9 g
Fibre	7.6 g
Starch	0.4 g
Sugars	16.5 g
Fat	221 g
Water	666 ml

Sunday's Dish of the Day
Berry Nice Chicken Salad

The weekend is a great time to relax and enjoy food with friends. This dish works really well when the meat is cooked on the barbecue as it can be eaten when the meat is still warm.

Ingredients for 1

75g or 3oz chicken breast halves

75g or 3oz mixed salad greens of the day

50g or 2oz of sugar snap peas

15g or half an oz of fresh blueberries

15g or half an oz of fresh raspberries

8 g or a third of an oz of toasted pecan nuts

90 mL or 6 tablespoons of peanut oil (save a little bit for grilling the chicken)

30 mL or 2 tablespoonfuls of cider vinegar

10 mL 2 teaspoons of honey

10 mL 2 teaspoons of fresh orange juice

Optional - A sprinkle of herbs to Provence

Preparations before you go...

Take a glass jar with a tight fitting lid (and old jam jar is ideal) and add the honey, vinegar, peanut oil, orange juice and a sprinkle of salt and pepper. Close the lid tightly and shake well.

Preheat your grill to high heat and lightly oil and grilled the chicken for 7 to 8 minutes on each side or until the juices run clear. Set to one side and allowed to cool then cut into strips.

Eating!

Take your snack box dish and put in the salad greens, blueberries, raspberries, peas, and pecan nuts add the chicken strips and mix a little then add the dressing to taste and toss thoroughly to coat the ingredients. Sprinkle over a few herbs if you like them.

If you're eating this freshly cooked. Mix the salad, add half the dressing and toss thoroughly. Let the meat cool slightly and then lay it over the top of the salad and pour over the rest of the dressing.

Staples for Today:

Salmon Tinned - 1 small tin
Beef Slices 3 x 50g (2oz) each
Chicken Breast 3 x 50g (2oz) Slices
Wensleydale x 50g (2oz)
Beaufort x 75g (3oz)f
American Cheese x 75g (3oz)

Mixed Salad 100g (4oz)
Tomatoes x 2 medium
Dill Pickle x 6
Sauce or Dip of choice x 20g
Pecan Nuts 50g (2oz)
Blueberries 25g (1 oz)
Fromage Blanche x 125g (5oz)

Nutrition for Today:

Protein	136.9 g
Carbs	56.9 g
Fibre	15.7 g
Starch	0.2 g
Sugars	30.6 g
Fat	237.7 g
Water	1069 ml

Nutrition for Week Three – Recap...

If you have managed to eat everything in the menus and on the staples lists for the third week of getting in shape - then you will have had a daily average of the following ...

Protein	183.2 g
Carbs	47.6 g
Fiber	12.9 g
Fat	191.6 g
Saturated	74.4 g
Omega-3	2.6 g
Omega-6	20.6 g
Cholesterol	610 mg

So Well done yet again! You have sped through your third week on the Snack Box Diet.

Don't forget to go and measure yourself again to see how you have progressed.

15.Menu Week Four

Monday

Dish of the Day - Tasty Broccoli Coleslaw

Tuesday

Dish of the Day - Cheesy Bacon and broccoli Salad

Wednesday

Dish of the Day – Smoked Sausage Salad

Thursday

Dish of the Day – Smoked Herring and Peppers in Mustard
Sauce

Friday

Dish of the Day - Italian Beef, Artichokes and Carrots Frappee

Saturday

Dish of the Day - Chicken Sausage, Apple Salad and Cooks
Dressing

Sunday

Dish of the Day - Spicy Taiwanese Beef Salad

Monday's Dish of the Day
Tasty Broccoli Coleslaw

I love coleslaw! It reminds me of parties, weddings and other family occasions. But most of all it reminds me of my mum as she was the one who taught me how to make it so many years ago. This is a variation on a theme and frankly you can add any tasty vegetables you like from the OK list and adjust the dressing as you see fit.

Ingredients for 1

2 slices of crispy bacon, crumble or chopped
50g or 2oz of green cabbage, roughly shredded
50g or 2oz of broccoli broken into its small florets
10g of sultanas or raisins
15g or half an oz of cashew nuts
10g of onions, roughly chopped
30g or 2 generous tablespoons of mayonnaise (more if you need it)
Salt and pepper to taste

Preparations before you leave ...

Fry or grill the bacon and allow to cool. In a medium-sized bowl mix together the bacon, green cabbage, broccoli, sultanas, cashew nuts and onion. Sprinkle over a little salt and pepper and dollop on the mayonnaise. Mix thoroughly, cover and leave in the refrigerator overnight. Transfer to your SnackBox when you're ready.

Eating!

You can add a little more mayonnaise just before eating if you think it's a little dry. Otherwise, just enjoy .

100

Staples for Today:

Beef and Pork/Danish Salami
  - 100g (4oz)
Chicken Leg x 2 Great with
  Coleslaw
Sardines in Oil x 1 small tin
Swiss x 75g (3oz)
Gouda x 75g (3oz)
Camembert x 75g (3oz)

Watercress 100g (4oz)
Peppers Green x half
Onions x 50g (2oz) - Salad or
  red as you prefer
Sauce or Dip of choice x 20g
Macadamia 50g (2oz)
Peach Fresh Small x1
  Fromage Blanche x 50g (2oz)

TIP:

You have bacon a few times this week so why not cook it all at once and save some time.

Nutrition for Today:

Protein	169.7 g
Carbs	54.4 g
Fibre	11.8 g
Starch	1.5g
Sugars	29.7 g
Fat	198.6 g
Water	768 ml

Tuesday's Dish of the Day
Cheesy Bacon and Broccoli Salad

Bacon and   cheese. Cheese and Onion - are wonderful combinations but as a trio - the tastes and textures combine so brilliantly that you need the broccoli to calm them down a bit.

Ingredients for 1

2 slices of bacon, well cooked and chopped roughly

12 broccoli florets

15g or half an oz of strong cheddar cheese - grated

15g or half an oz of red onion chopped or sliced into fine rings

5 mL or 1 teaspoonfuls of red wine vinegar

Half teaspoonfull of honey (optional)

15 mL or 1 tablespoon of mayonnaise

Squeeze of lemon juice

Salt and pepper to taste

Preparation before you leave...

Grill or fry the bacon, allow to cool and then chop or crumble.

To make the dressing. In a small glass jar with a tight fitting lid add the red wine vinegar, mayonnaise, lemon juice, salt and pepper. Shake together nicely.

Eating!

In your snack box diet bowl, add the chopped bacon, broccoli florets, cheddar cheese and onion rings. Pour over the dressing, mix well and leave for 10 to 15 minutes before enjoying.

Staples for Today:

Chicken Legs x 2
Sardines in Oil x 1 small tin
Pate - 50g (2oz) Nice country
   one or to your own taste
Cheddar x 50g (2oz)
Leerdammer x 50g (2oz)
Baby Swiss x 75g (3oz)

Endives - 100g (4oz)
Tomatoes x 2 medium
Radishes x 9
Sauce or Dip of choice x 20g
Peanuts 50g (2oz)
Yogurt Greek 125g (5oz)

Nutrition for Today:

Protein	160.7 g
Carbs	47.2 g
Fibre	14.7 g
Starch	0.5 g
Sugars	18.2 g
Fat	176 g
Water	940 ml

SNACK BOX DIET

Wednesday's Dish of the Day
Smoked Sausage Salad

This is a super dish which is also called burnt sausage salad in our house. The idea of cooking the sausages well is to get that slightly smoky flavour and that of course means that it goes well with any smoked sausage you care to use. (Or any burnt ones for that matter)

Ingredients for 1

45 ml or 3 tablespoons olive oil

2 or 3 turkey sausages

half a Granny Smith apple

100g or 4oz of mixed salad leaves

2 small spring onions, cleaned and finely sliced

Half celery stick cut into 1cm pieces

30 mL or 2 tablespoons of lemon juice

15g or half oz of pecan nuts

15g or half oz blue cheese this

3 mL or half a teaspoon of Dijon mustard

Preparation before you go ...

Pour 15 mL or one tablespoon of the olive oil into a skillet or frying pan and fry the sausages until they are very well done - brown to almost black in some places. (But obviously not cremated). Allow to cool, then cut into 1 cm rings.

Pour the rest of the olive oil into a screw top jar add in the lemon juice, Dijon mustard and salt and pepper, close firmly and shake well until the sauce is nice and creamy.

Eating!

Place the salad greens into a bowl, add in the spring onions, celery, pecan nuts, blue cheese, half of the dressing and toss well. Lay the sausages and apples over the top then pour on the rest of the dressing.

Staples for Today:

Sardines in Oil x 1 small tin
Pate - 50g (2oz)
Turkey Sausages x 6 x 20g
   Well cooked and sliced or
   cubed and added to the
   salad
Romano x 75g (3oz)
Mimolette x 75g (3oz)
Buxton Blue x 75g (3oz)
Escarole x 100g (4oz)

Celery x 2 sticks chopped in
   to 1cm slices if you prefer
Spring Onions - 50g (2oz)
Carrots Grated 50g (2oz)
Sauce or Dip of choice x 20g
Pecans 50g (2oz)
1 small apple
 Fromage Blanche x 50g (2oz)

Nutrition for Today:

Protein	122.7 g
Carbs	48.5 g
Fibre	14.7 g
Starch	1.2 g
Sugars	24.2 g
Fat	158.7 g
Water	591 ml

Thursday's Dish of the Day - Smoked Herring and Peppers in Mustard Sauce

This is a tasty one! Of course you can use any smoked fish with this recipe – it seems to work fine for all of them. You can also add in other ingredients from the OK list if you fancy a bit of a change.

Ingredients for 1

1 boneless smoked herring fillet	15 L or 1 tablespoon of olive oil
100g or 1 cup of mixed salad	15 mL or 1 tablespoon of cider vinegar (white wine vinegar will do)
1 egg	
Half sweet red pepper, sliced or diced	Healthy Pinch of dried tarragon
15 mL or 1 tablespoon of Dijon mustard	Salt and Pepper to Taste

Preparation before you go ...

Hardball the egg, allow to cool and peel it.

Pour the olive oil into a glass jar with a firmly closing lid, add the cider vinegar, mustard, tarragon, and a good pinch of salt and pepper.

Eating!

Place the salad on your plate and break the herring fillet over the top. Quarter or slice the egg and add that to the dish then pour the dressing over the top, quantity according to your own taste.

Staples for Today:

Pate - 50g (2oz) Nice country
   one or to your own taste
Turkey Sausages x 6 x 20gr
Herring Smoked 1 Boneless
   Fillet
Monterey Jack x 50g (2oz)
   Dry x 50g (2oz)
Cheese Muenster x 50g (2oz)
Curd x 50g (2oz)

Alfalfa sprouts 50g (2oz)
Tomatoes x 2 medium
Peppers Red x half
Sauce or Dip of choice x 20g
Pine-nuts 50g (2oz)
Natural live yogurt x 1 pot
   125gr (5oz)

Nutrition for Today:

Protein	115.5 g
Carbs	33.1 g
Fibre	7.3 g
Starch	0.7 g
Sugars	21.1 g
Fat	146.6 g
Water	759 ml

Friday's Dish of the Day - Italian Beef, Artichokes and Carrots Râpées

Finely cut Italian beef is quite moorish and I can eat it like candy – well up to a point. When you add in the artichoke hearts and carrot and you have a very nice meal for little effort

Ingredients for 1

100g or 4oz of dry Italian beef
2 marinated artichoke hearts
100g or 4oz of spinach, torn
6 Cherry tomatoes, quartered
50g or 2oz of grated carrot
45 ml or three tablespoons of groundnut oil

15 mL or 1 tablespoon of cider vinegar
5 mL or 1 teaspoon of Dijon mustard
Healthy Pinch of, dried basil leaves
Salt and pepper to taste

Preparations before you go ...

Pour the groundnut oil into a sealable glass jar add the cider vinegar, Dijon mustard and basil leaves and shake vigorously.

Cut the sliced beef into strips and quarter the artichokes.

Eating!

Spread the spinach over your plate and place the grated carrot in the centre. Lay the beef strips over the top and decorate with the quartered artichokes and tomatoes. Pour over the dressing and enjoy.

108

Staples for Today:

Turkey Sausages x 6 x 20g
Herring Smoked 1 Fillet
Beef Dry Italian 150g (6oz)
    Or...Cut into chunks, dice
    pepper add some olives
    and salad leaves cover with
    french dressing
Leicester x 75g (3oz)
Port Salut x 50g (2oz)
Brie x 75g (3oz)

Spinach leaves x 100g (4oz)
Chives - 20g - Chopped fine
    and mixed with fish or other
    salad
Olives Green x 20
Sauce or Dip of choice x 20g
Pistachios 50g (2oz)
Apple x 1
Fromage Blanche x 50g (2oz)

Nutrition for Today:

Protein	152 g
Carbs	57.2 g
Fibre	17.6 g
Starch	1.8 g
Sugars	29 g
Fat	174.7 g
Water	661 ml

Saturday's Dish of the Day - Chicken Sausage, Apple Salad and Cooks Dressing

I really love fruit and meat together. This recipe has a curious twist in that the dressing is made from warm ingredients and allow to cool. Delicious!

Ingredients for 1

2 or 3 chicken sausages sliced in half lengthwise
100g or 4oz of mixed salad greens
6 Cherry tomatoes, halved
30 ml or 2 tablespoons of

lemon juice
30 ml or 2 tablespoons of olive oil
5 ml or 1 teaspoon of mustard
5 ml or 1 teaspoon of honey
Salt and pepper to taste

Preparations before you go ...

Add 15 ml or one tablespoon of the olive oil to a heavy bottomed frying pan or skillet and cook the sausages and till well browned. Take the pan off the heat, remove the sausages and allow them to cool and then cut into 1 cm pieces.

Add the lemon juice honey and mustard to the pan and combine that with the juices from the sausages. Whisk in the rest of the olive oil and then set aside to cool totally then pour into a sealable glass jar. Adding salt and pepper to taste.

Eating!

Add the mixed greens to your plate or bowl add in the sausages and cherry tomatoes. Pour over the cooks dressing and enjoy.

Staples for Today:

Herring Smoked 1 Fillet –
   Add a few olives and eat
   with the salad with a light
   dressing
Beef Dry Italian x 150g (6oz)
Chicken Sausages x 6 x 20g -
   Well cooked and sliced
Lancashire x 50g (2oz)
Roquefort x 50g (2oz)

Dauphin x 50g (2oz)
Lettuce x 100g (4oz)
Tomatoes Sun-Dried 125g
   (5oz)
Olives Black x 20
Sauce or Dip of choice x 20g
Pumpkin seeds 50g (2oz)
Yogurt Greek 125g (5oz)

If you are having the dish of the day at home, you can have it with the sausages still warm - that's tasty too!

Nutrition for Today:

Protein	131.3 g
Carbs	54.9 g
Fibre	16.1 g
Starch	0.4 g
Sugars	24.2 g
Fat	151.1 g
Water	560 ml

Sunday's Dish of the Day
Spicy Taiwanese Beef Salad

I've put this one on the weekend as it may be you'd like to have something a bit different. If your eating it straight away you can have it so the meat is warm and if you want to share with a friend – just multiply the ingredients accordingly.

Ingredients for 1

125g or 5 oz steak fillet

4 lettuce leaves - washed and torn bite-size pieces

50g or 2oz of cucumber, diced

6 cherry tomatoes

1 spring onion chopped finely

30g or half a cup of lemon grass cut into centimetre pieces

15g where half an oz of fresh chopped coriander leaves

(cilantro)

5g or quarter oz of fresh mint leaves

45 ml or 3 tablespoons of lime juice

10 ml 2 teaspoons of fish sauce

3 ml or half a teaspoon of sweet chilli sauce

One spoon of honey

Preparation before you leave ...

Preheat the grill to high heat.

To make the sauce. In a medium bowl stir together the lime juice, fish sauce, chilli sauce, and honey. Add in the green onions, lemon grass, mint leaves, coriander, and stir until well mixed. Set to one side.

Cook the steak for 4 to 5 minutes on each side until it is cooked to no more than medium. Remove, and slice into thin strips. Allow to cool a little and then add the meat juices to the sauce you made earlier and add in the meat. Stir a little so the meat is covered by the sauce then cover tightly and refrigerate.

112

Eating:

Put the lettuce into your snack box diet bowl, throw on the cucumber and then pour over the meat and sauce, top off with cherry tomatoes and an artistically placed coriander leaf or two.

Staples for Today:

Beef Dry Italian x 150gr
Chicken Sausages x 6 x 20gr
Tuna in Brine x 1 small tin -
    Just dip into it as you want
    or mix with salad
Jarlsberg x 75g (3oz)
Saint-Paulin x 75g (3oz)
Boursin x 75g (3oz)
Lettuce Iceberg x100g (4oz)

Cucumber x 50g (2oz)
Fennel – Finochio half
    medium bulb
Cherry Tomatoes x 10
Sauce or Dip of choice x 20g
Sesame seeds 50g (2oz)
Orange x1
    Fromage Blanche x 50g (2oz)

Nutrition for Today:

Protein	203.8 g
Carbs	62.4 g
Fibre	15.3 g
Starch	0.6 g
Sugars	24.3 g
Fat	149.7 g
Water	920 ml

113

Nutrition for Week Four – Recap...

If you have got through everything in the menus and on the staples lists for the forth week of getting in shape - then you will have had a daily average of the following ...

Protein	150.8 g
Carbs	51.1 g
Fiber	13.9 g
Fat	165.1 g
Saturated	58.3 g
Omega-3	2.4 g
Omega-6	22.3 g
Cholesterol	577 mg

So Well done yet again! You have torn through your forth week on the Snack Box Diet.

Don't forget to go and measure yourself again to see how you have progressed.

16. MENU WEEK FIVE

Monday

Dish of the Day - Sausage, Egg and Apple Salad

Tuesday

Dish of the Day - Traditional Salad Nicoise

Wednesday

Dish of the Day – Corned Beef in Thousand Islands Dressing and Nutty Croutons

Thursday

Dish of the Day – Chicken and Dill Salad

Friday

Dish of the Day - Smoked Salmon in a Tomato Vinaigrette

Saturday

Dish of the Day - Deli-cious Crab Salad

Sunday

Dish of the Day - Cold Meats and Creamy Mushrooms

Monday's Dish of the Day
Sausage, Egg and Apple Salad

Although it might sound like a strange combination - this salad is absolutely delicious. And of course, you can have any sausage you like to use. I do find however that I prefer the sausages well cooked.

Ingredients for 1

1 hard-boiled egg, roughly chopped

1 the well cooked sausage, cubed or sliced

15g or half an oz of Gruyère cheese, grated

Quarter of an Apple, chopped

5g or one tablespoon of chopped parsley

2 or 3 lettuce leaves, torn into bite-size pieces.

Dressing

15 ml or 1 tablespoon full of peanut oil

5 ml or 1 teaspoon of cider vinegar

Quarter teaspoon of Dijon mustard

A pinch of paprika

Salt and pepper to taste

Preparations before you go...

Put all the ingredients for the dressing in a glass jar with a tight fitting lid and shake until well blended.

Eating!

Put all the main ingredients into your bowl and mix well. Pour over dressing, mix again and enjoy. Don't chop the apple until your ready to eat or will discolour.

Staples for Today:

Chicken Sausages 6 x 20gr	Monastery Cheeses 50g (2oz)
Tuna in Brine x1 tin	Lettuce 100g (4oz)
Beef Corned 100g (4oz) Sliced	Romaine 100g (4oz)
- goes great with tomatoes	Tomatoes 2 medium
and cheese	Dill Pickle x 6
Gruyère 50g (2oz)	Sauce or Dip of choice 20g
Canadian Cheddar 75g (3oz)	Sunflower seeds 50g (2oz)
75g (3oz)	Natural live yogurt 1 pot 125g

Nutrition for Today:

Protein	139 g
Carbs	51.8 g
Fibre	14.9 g
Starch	0 g
Sugars	27.3 g
Fat	143.8 g
Water	1110 ml

117

Tuesday's Dish of the Day
Traditional Salade Niçoise

It has to be said that there are numerous versions of this salad from Provence in France. Yet all of them have the same basic ingredients including eggs, lettuce, tomatoes, anchovies and olives. It does take a little longer than most dishes to prepare but sometimes you do deserve something a little special.

Ingredients for 1

1 hard-boiled egg,

1 large firm tomato,

50g or 2oz of French beans

Half an onion, sliced into fine rings

4 generous lettuce leaves, shredded

Quarter of a green/red pepper, seeded and cut into thin strips lengthwise.

25g or 1oz of tuna, in oil or brine as you prefer. Drained, ready to use

4 anchovy fillets

8 or 10 black olives

For the dressing

30 ml or 2 tablespoons of groundnut oil

15 ml or 1 table spoon of cider vinegar (red wine vinegar works)

Quarter teaspoon of French mustard

Healthy pinch of salt and pepper

1 clove of garlic, chopped fine or crushed

Preparations before you go...

Hard-boiled eggs for 8 to 10 minutes, cool, shell and quarter them.

Top and tail the French beans and cook in boiling water for 6 to 8 minutes, drain and set aside to cool. Put all ingredients for the dressing in a sealable glass jar and shake until you have a smooth and creamy sauce.

118

Eating!

Put the shredded lettuce leaves and French beans into your bowl and pour over half the French dressing and toss thoroughly. Pile the tuna into the middle of the salad and arrange the anchovy's coming out like the spokes on a wheel. Add the olives peppers and onion rings, tomatoes and hard-boiled eggs. Pour over the rest of the dressing allowed to stand for a minute or two and then enjoy.

Staples for Today:

Tuna in Brine x1 tin
Beef Corned 100g (4oz)
Chicken Breast 3 x 50g (2oz)
  Slices
Grafton Village Cheddar 75g
  (3oz)
Cantal 75g (3oz)
Bath Cheese 50g (2oz)
Mustard and Cress 50g (2oz)

Peppers Green x half
Onions 50g (2oz) - Salad or
  red as you prefer
Beetroot 50g (2oz) sliced or
  cubed
Walnuts 50g (2oz)
Apricot Fresh x1
 Fromage Blanche 50g (2oz)

Nutrition for Today:

Protein	142.2 g
Carbs	38.9 g
Fibre	9.9 g
Starch	0.2 g
Sugars	18.5 g
Fat	157.6 g
Water	689 ml

119

Wednesday's Dish of the Day - Corned Beef, Thousand Islands Dressing & Nutty Croutons

Corned beef does not have to be boring - and this dish proves it! Just try it - you'll see what I mean. And anyway, who said thousand island dressing is only mean for shrimps or prawns?

Ingredients for 1

50g or 2oz of corned beef, in 1 cm cubes

100g or 4oz of iceberg lettuce, ripped into bite sized chunks

1 spring onion, the white sliced into fine rings and 2 or 3 cm of the stalk finely chopped

1 hard-boiled egg, roughly chopped

25g or 1oz of parsley, roughly chopped

45 ml or 3 tablespoons of mayonnaise

15 ml or 1 table spoon of tomato ketchup

15g or half an oz of lightly chopped walnuts

5 ml or 1 teaspoon of pickled relish (virtually any type)

Dash of Worcestershire sauce

salt and pepper to taste

Preparations before you go...

In a suitable bowl mix together the mayonnaise, tomato ketchup, egg, spring onion rings, Worcestershire sauce and relish. Add salt and pepper to taste. Transfer the mixture into a screw top jar and place in the refrigerator to cool..

Eating!

Toss together the lettuce, spring onion green bits and corned beef. Pour over the dressing and mix well then top off with the walnuts.

120

Staples for Today:

Beef Corned 100g (4oz) Sliced
  - goes great with tomatoes
  and cheese
Chicken Breast 3 x 50g (2oz)
  Slices
Smoked Salmon 100g (4oz)
  Slices
Emmental 50g (2oz)
Cheddar 75g (3oz)
Reblochon 50g (2oz)

Parsley - 50g (2oz)
Tomatoes 2 medium
Radishes x 9
Sauce or Dip of choice x 20g
Almonds Roasted 50g (2oz)
Yogurt Greek
Roasted almonds go with both
  chicken and salmon – add a
  little french dressing too if
  you like it.

Nutrition for Today:

Protein	136.3 g
Carbs	44.2 g
Fibre	14.5 g
Starch	1.7 g
Sugars	17.6 g
Fat	125.2 g
Water	777 ml

Thursday's Dish of the Day
Chicken and Dill Salad

An absolutely simple dish to make. And refreshing too. You can use lime in place of the lemon if you want a change - I like it with either one.

Ingredients for 1

1 small chicken breast
1 Hard-Boiled Egg Chopped
1 Large Dill pickle chopped
1 Spring Onion trimmed and chopped
75 ml or 5 tablespoons of mayonnaise
75 ml or 5 tablespoonfuls of soured cream
1 teaspoon of drained capers
2 teaspoons of fresh dill chopped
15g or half an oz of pecan nuts
A squeeze of lemon for a bit of bite
Salt-and-pepper to taste

Preparation before you go ...

Lightly oil the chicken breast and grill or fry for 5 to 7 minutes on each side or until the juices run clear. Allow to cool and cut into strips then cover and refrigerate.

Eating!

Put all ingredients in your snack box bowl and toss well. Squeeze the lemon juice over the top.

Staples for Today:

Chicken Breast 3 x 50g (2oz)
   Cut into strips or sliced
Smoked Salmon 75g (3oz)
   Slices
Beef Salami 100g (4oz)
Dutch Mimolette 75g (3oz)
Cheshire 50g (2oz)
Babybel x 4
Roquette 100g (4oz)

Celery 2 sticks chopped in to
   1cm slices if you prefer
Spring Onions - 50g (2oz)
Sauce or Dip of choice x 20g
Brazil nuts 50g (2oz)
Blueberries Fresh 70g or half
   cup
  Fromage Blanche 50g (2oz)

Tip:

You can use ready cooked chicken breast if you want but sometimes home cooked one have a much nicer taste.

Nutrition for Today:

Protein	122.3 g
Carbs	46.1 g
Fibre	12.7 g
Starch	2.9 g
Sugars	23.8 g
Fat	208.8 g
Water	771 ml

Friday's Dish of the Day
Smoked Salmon in a Tomato Vinaigrette

Some think it's bad form to put smoked salmon in tomato vinaigrette - that is until they try it. I'll let you decide whether you like it or not.

Ingredients for 1

100g or 4oz of smoked salmon, cut into strips
100g or 4oz of salad greens
1 hard-boiled egg, sliced
Half a small red pepper, de-seeded and sliced lengthwise
30 ml or 2 tablespoons of tomato ketchup
30 ml or 2 tablespoons of olive oil
30 ml or 2 tablespoons of cider vinegar
3 ml or half a teaspoon of honey
A good pinch of dried oregano, dried basil and garlic powder

Preparation before you go ...

Apart from hard-boiling the egg you just need to make the dressing. Put the ketchup, oil, vinegar, honey, oregano, basil and garlic powder in a small glass jar and shake until thoroughly combined and you have a nice creamy sauce.

Eating!

Arrange the salad greens on your plate, arrange the salmon, egg and red pepper slices over the top and simply pour the dressing - as much or as little as you desire.

Staples for Today:

Smoked Salmon 75g (3oz)
  Slices
Beef Salami 100g (4oz)
Turkey Drum Sticks x 2 Just
  eat off the bone
Double Worcester 50g
(2oz)
Devon Blue 50g (2oz)
Tomme de Chevre 75g
(3oz)

Sorrel 100g (4oz)
Tomatoes 2 medium or 50g
  (2oz)
Chives - 25g (1oz) - Chopped
  fine and mixed with fish or
  other salad
Sauce or Dip of choice x 20g
Cashews 50g (2oz)
Natural live yogurt 125g (5oz)

Nutrition for Today:

Protein	218.6 g
Carbs	50.4 g
Fibre	7.9 g
Starch	0 g
Sugars	23.6 g
Fat	191.5g
Water	958 ml

Saturday's Dish of the Day
Deli-cious Crab Salad

This recipe has the 'fresh from the deli' taste that just can not be beaten. As it's the weekend, you may want to make more and share with some friends.

Ingredients for 1

100g or 4oz of crabmeat
Aalf a red pepper, cleaned and diced
a quarter of a small red onion, finely sliced
Half a celery stick cut into 1 cm pieces
30 ml or 2 tablespoons of mayonnaise

5 ml or 1 teaspoon of salad cream
5 ml or 1 teaspoon of lemon juice
A good pinch of oregano
3 ml or half a teaspoon of red wine vinegar
Salt and pepper to taste.

Preparations before you go ...

Mix together the mayonnaise, soured cream, lemon juice, oregano, vinegar and salt and pepper. Spoon into a screw top jar and set aside.

Eating!

Put the crab into a bowl and break up with a fork. Add the onions, green peppers and celery and combine thoroughly.

Pour over the dressing and toss lightly.

Tip: Keep all ingredients in the refrigerator before serving or mix together, cover and chill an hour or two before you want to eat it.

126

Staples for Today:

Beef Salami 100g (4oz)
Turkey Drum Sticks x 1 Just
eat off the bone
Crab Meat - 1 small tin or
cooked fresh 100g (4oz)
Broken up and mixed with
salad
Dorset Blue 50g (2oz)
Double Gloucester 50g (2oz)
Truffe 50g (2oz)

Watercress 100g (4oz)
Peppers Red small
Olives Green x 20
Sauce or Dip of choice x 20g
Coconut Dried Sliced 50g
(2oz)
Blueberries Fresh 50g (2oz)
ams or half small cup
Fromage Blanche 50g (2oz)

Nutrition for Today:

Protein	183 g
Carbs	38.2 g
Fibre	10.6 g
Starch	1.1 g
Sugars	18.4 g
Fat	168.9 g
Water	820 ml

Sunday's Dish of the Day
Cold Meats and Creamy Mushrooms

This dish has an echo of beef stroganoff to it - but obviously is meant to be eaten cold.

Ingredients for 1

75g or 3oz of thinly sliced cold meat or poultry
60 ml or 4 tablespoons of double cream
5 ml or 1 teaspoon of lemon juice
50g or 1oz of sliced mushrooms
1 small carrot, grated
A small bunch of watercress
6 to 10 slices of cucumber
3 or 4 lettuce leaves, shredded
A good pinch of nutmeg
Salt and pepper

Preparations before you go ...

Mix the cream and lemon juice and then pour in the mushrooms and carrots. Add a pinch or two of nutmeg and season with salt and pepper.

Eating!

Put a ring of watercress and shredded lettuce around the edge of the plate, roll up the meat into tubes and place them inside of the lettuce leaving space in the middle to pile in the mushroom mixture. Arrange the cucumber artistically - or not - as you see fit.

Staples for Today:

Turkey Drum Sticks x 1 Just
  eat off the bone
Crab Meat - 1 small tin or 75g
  (3oz)
Ham Slices - 3 x 50g (2oz) -
  Filled with Soft cheese of
  choice and rolled
Derby 75g (3oz)
Gloucester 50g (2oz)
Pepper Jack 50g (2oz)

Endives - 100g (4oz)
Mushrooms - 6 medium
  chopped or sliced fine
Fennel – Finochio half
  medium bulb
Couscous 50g (2oz)– Nice
  with the fish
Sauce or Dip of choice x 20g
Coconut Fresh 50g (2oz)
Yogurt Greek 125g (5oz)

Nutrition for Today:

Protein	224.8 g
Carbs	50.3 g
Fibre	15.5 g
Starch	1.2 g
Sugars	9.4 g
Fat	130.5 g
Water	1013 ml

Nutrition for Week Five – Recap...

If you eat everything in the menus and on the staples lists for the fifth week of finding who you really are underneath - then you will have had a daily average of the following ...

Protein	166.6 g
Carbs	45.7 g
Fiber	12.3 g
Fat	160.9 g
Saturated	61.6 g
Omega-3	2.9 g
Omega-6	22.4 g
Cholesterol	592 mg

So Well done yet again! You have torn through your fifth and last official week on the Snack Box Diet.

Don't forget to go and measure yourself again to see how you have progressed.

From now on you can go back to the first week and start again or have a look at the website www.SnackBoxDiet.com for more ideas.

17. PRACTICAL TIPS

Advice on Quantities

Most of the time the amount of food that you get each day should be more than adequate for you. Remember this is not a contest so you do not have to eat everything that's allocated for that day.

If you're not hungry don't eat it!

If you are following the diet properly, you should notice that by the time you have been on the diet for two or three weeks that you will not be eating everything on the list for each day anyway. I know for myself I probably eat half the quantity that is listed down for each day and I'm still more than satisfied.

Remember, one of the advantages of eating foods that are more satisfying is that they take longer to digest. This in turn means your stomach becomes empty less quickly which in turn means you won't want to eat so soon.

That means that your stomach will get gradually smaller until it returns to its appropriate size.

On the other hand if when you first start the diet, you find you are not quite satisfied with the amount of food that is given each day. Then you are more than welcome to add as many of the free to eat ingredients on the OK list as you want.

But if you're still doing that after weeks three or week four at the latest - well that's OK provided your measurements are getting smaller. If your measurements are not getting smaller then it's time to admit your a bit of a pig and so should exercise some self control.

Remember, these quantities are more than enough for a man of 175 cm and weighing 83 kg (5'9" at 183lbs).

Who by most systems would be (depending on frame size) classed as 7 to 10 kg or 15 to 20 lbs over weight!

Long Term Use of The Snack Box Diet

I've been eating this type of food for years and can only say that in general, my health is very good. I have never needed a doctor all the time I've been eating this way - I guess that says something.

In essence the five week plan in this book is all about teaching your body to get used to eating healthier foods and retraining your mind to not see food as a crutch or substitute but simply as nutrition. Something good and wholesome that should be enjoyable to eat.

Certainly, once you are more adept at making good food choices this training will allow you to add in a greater range of food and also, to know when you have had enough of something and the strength to say 'no!' And not go back for more.

Notes on Recipes

Nothing is written in stone as far as recipes go - remember they are a guide. And no matter what recipe you come to, you can always adapt it slightly to suit your own tastes and the ingredients you have to hand. Sometimes, ingredients can be exchanged, added in or left out entirely. That really is up to you.

However, I would recommend that the first time you try a recipe you follow the ingredients I've put down and then adapt it to your own taste once you know what it should taste like - according to my taste anyway.

As far as quantities go, remember the dish of the day is actually in addition to the staples for each day. Although where appropriate I have used some of the foods listed on the staples ingredients within the recipe for that day.

However, it is important that you follow either the metric or the non-metric measurements. That's mainly because there are differences between the quantities. For instance as far as tablespoons go the standard British tablespoon holds 17.7 ml. The US tablespoon is 14.2 ml while the Australian tablespoon is 20 ml. So use whichever one you are comfortable with but make sure you stick with that one and don't switch backwards and forwards.

Realistically though, I don't suppose it would matter too much except where you get onto some of the more powerful/tasty ingredients.

Italian Dressing

45ml or 3 tablespoons olive oil

15ml or 1 tablespoons white wine vinegar

10g or 1 tablespoon chopped fresh parsley

10ml or 2 teaspoons fresh lemon juice

1 garlic cloves, chopped

2g 1 teaspoon dried basil, crumbled

Good pinch dried crushed red pepper

Pinch of dried oregano

Make at least 8 hours ahead to allow the flavours to infuse. Combine all ingredients in a bowl and whisk together. Add Salt and Pepper to taste. You can make more if you want as it keeps well in the refrigerator.

18. DESSERTS

You may be wondering "What can I have as a dessert on this diet?" Well within reason you can have anything that is not high is sugar or other carbohydrates. So things like sorbets, traditionally made cheesecakes, nut based cakes, cream based egg custards and more.

The only thing I would say is not to have anything with artificial sweeteners in - Full Stop. Use honey, or stevia to sweeten things up and also get used to not eating so many sugary things - they really aren't that good for you at all anyway.

Stevia in the form of extract, powder, liquid or dried leaves can be bought from most good quality health food shops and from many online retailers. You can even grow your own!

Though if you have a little time to make something - here are some suggestions for when you fancy something sweet.

There will be more on www.SnackBoxDiet.com

Cream Brulee

400ml or 14 fl oz Cream
4 egg yolks
1 egg white
8 packets stevia extract

3 or 4 teaspoons vanilla
 extract
Cocoa powder

Pour the cream into the top half of a large double boiler or into a bowl over a pan of boiling water. Whisk in the egg yolks so no streaks remain, then whisk in the egg white.

 Add the stevia and the vanilla extract.

Continue cooking until the mixture thickens enough to coat the back of a spoon and a custard type mixture is obtained.

Pour into a souffle dish or individual ramekins and allow to cool. Move to refrigerator and cool for at least 3 to 4 hours. Just before serving, dust each one with a little cocoa powder or dust with demerara sugar and flame to caramelise the sugar. As an alternative, you can put a few of your permitted fruits in the ramekin before you pour in the mixture.

Should give about 6 to 8 servings

Nutrition per Serving:

Protein	22.9 g
Carbs	14.3 g
Fibre	15.5 g
Starch	0 g
Sugars	101 g
Fat	172.5 g
Water	305 ml

Fruity Muffins

225g or 9oz Almond Flour
60g or 2 1/2 oz Butter - melted
4 Eggs
1 g or 2 teaspoons baking
  powder
1/2 teaspoon stevia extract

1g or 1/4 teaspoon salt
75ml or 5 tablespoons of
  water
Fruit of your choice, small
  piece

Preheat oven to 180C and grease a 12 muffin tin. Mix all the dry ingredients together in a large bowl. Beat the eggs and turn into the dry ingredients, add in the water and mix thoroughly. Spoon the mixture into the muffin tin half filling the moulds then bake for 15 minutes.

Obviously makes 12 delicious muffins.

Tip: you can put either blueberries, fruit or a half teaspoon of jam on each muffin before you bake them for an extra treat.

Nutrition per Serving/Muffin:

Protein	6 g
Carbs	3.2 g
Fibre	2 g
Starch	0 g
Sugars	1 g
Fat	15 g
Water	20 ml

Spicy Pecans Bakes

0.5g 1/4 teaspoon nutmeg

1g or1/4 teaspoon ground
  clove

2.5 g or teaspoon cinnamon

4 g or 3/4 teaspoon salt

1 egg white

200g or 8 oz pecans

4 teaspoons stevia blend or 8
  packets of stevia

30 ml or 2 tablespoons water

Combine all spices and stevia in a bowl. In a second bowl, beat the egg white with water until bubbles form. Add the pecans to egg mixture and coat well. Spoon dollops of coated pecans on a greased baking sheet and sprinkle over the spice mixture. Bake at 150 C for 30-minutes. Allow to cool before serving.

Should make about 10 servings

Nutrition per Serving:

Protein	2.2 g
Carbs	3 g
Fibre	2 g
Starch	0.1 g
Sugars	1 g
Fat	14.5 g
Water	3 ml

No Bake Cheesecake

455g (1lb) cream cheese
1 package unflavoured
  gelatine
1 cup boiling water

15g or 5 teaspoons stevia
  powder blend.
3g or 1 teaspoon vanilla

Dissolve the gelatine into the boiling water in a large mixing bowl. Add in the cream cheese and vanilla and beat until light. Add the stevia and mix a bit more until light & fluffy. Spoon into dessert dishes and refrigerate for about 1 1/2 to 2 hours until set. Serve cold. Garnish with your permitted fruits, your favourite sauce or serve just as it is.

Should make about 8 Servings

Nutrition per Serving:

Protein	3.7 g
Carbs	2.5 g
Fibre	2 g
Starch	0.25 g
Sugars	2 g
Fat	21.4 g
Water	34 ml

Notes:

PART TWO

This is where the work starts!

"Don't wait until everything is just right. It will never be perfect. There will always be challenges, obstacles and less than perfect conditions. So what. Get started now. With each step you take, you will grow stronger and stronger, more and more skilled, more and more self-confident and more and more successful."

Mark Victor Hansen

19. YOUR PROGRESS LOGS

Step One

Taking your Measurements

Step Two

List of things fat stop me from having

List of Needs

My List of Wants

Personal Qualities I

Step One
How to fill in the
Measurement Tables.

Men Only

1. On the first day of your diet, measure each part of your body as shown in the mans diagram. Either in centimetres or inches.

2. Add up all those measurements and note that in the 'Total for Week' line directly below those measurements.

3. Weigh yourself and note that down too.

Look at those measurement and pick two or more and decide on a realistic amount you can lose in 5 – 6 weeks.

So, if say you started with a 45 inch waist - a realistic goal could be to get to 39 inches. Or you could put down the ultimate size you want to say 34 inches - do whatever you think will motivate you the most!

Do the same for at least one of the other measurements.

4. Note down your target sizes in the right hand column.

That's all you need to do for the first time. But...

5. On the same day the week after, take those measurements again, add them up and see how much you have lost.

6. Continue doing that each week there after - until you hit your goals.

144

Mens Measurements

Using the mens diagram take the following measurements...

1. Around your neck - Where a shirt collar would go.

2. Around your chest - Just under your armpits more or less at nipple level.

3. Stomach/Waist - At the largest part.

4. Upper arm - At the largest part of your upper arm, without flexing the muscles and your arms straight

5. Forearm - at the largest part of your forearm with your arms straight, without flexing the muscles.

6. Thighs - at the largest part of each leg measured separately

7. Calves - At the largest part of your calf

You can either measure both arms and legs then add them together (more accurate) or just pick one side and stick with it (quicker to do).

Don't worry that you haven't as many measurements as the ladies. Men and women not only put on weight differently, they also lose it differently too.

Measure each part of your body and note it down on the table. Use either centimetres or inches as you prefer – but keep to the same throughout the diet.

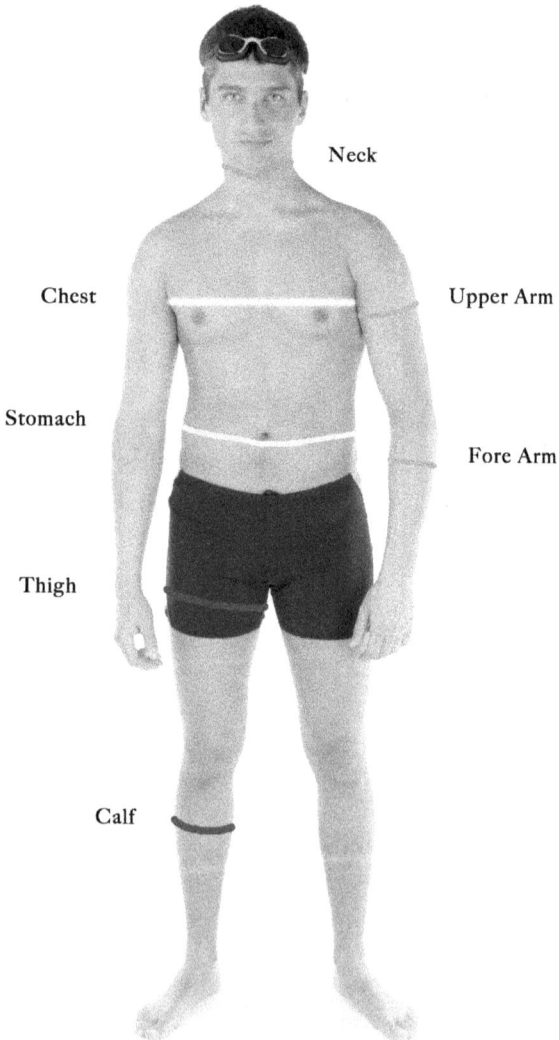

Neck

Chest

Upper Arm

Stomach

Fore Arm

Thigh

Calf

	First Day	End of Week 1	End of Week 2	End of Week 3	End of Week 5	Goal
Neck						
Chest						
Stomach						
Upper Arm						
Forearm						
Thigh						
Calf						
Total for Week						
Weight						

How to fill in the
Measurement Tables.

Ladies Only

1. On the first day of your diet, measure each part of your body as shown in the Ladies diagram. Either in centimetres or inches.

2. Add up all those measurements and note that in the 'Total for Week' line directly below your measurements.

3. Weigh yourself and note that down too.

Look at those measurement and pick two or more and decide on a realistic amount you an lose in 5 – 6 weeks.

So, if say you started with a 36 inch waist - a realistic goal could be to get to 32 inches. Or you could put down the ultimate size you want to say 26 inches - do whatever you think will motivate you the most!

The same goes for dress size. Decide on a realistic goal- say dropping two sizes or put in the ultimate (but realistic) goal your aiming for at the end of the diet.

Do the same for at least one of the other measurement.

4. Note down your target sizes in the right hand column.

That's all you need to do for this time...

5. On the same day the week after take those measurements again, add them up and see how much you have lost.

6. Continue doing that each week there after until you hit your goals.

Ladies Measurements

Using the ladies diagram take the following measurements...

1. **Around your neck** - Where a shirt collar would go.

2. **Chest** - Keeping the measuring tape parallel with the ground, measure around your bra directly under your bust after expelling all air from your lungs - you want this measurement to be as small as possible.

3. **Bust** - Standing straight, with your arms at your side, measure at the fullest part of your bust (while wearing a non-padded bra) making sure the measuring tape is parallel with the ground and not binding.

4. **Upper arm** - at the largest part of your upper arm, without flexing your muscles and your arms straight.

5. **Forearm** - at the largest part of your forearm with your arms straight and without flexing the muscles.

6. **Waist** - Ideally at the smallest part but you be the judge - just keep to the same place each week.

7. **Stomach** - At the largest part.

8. **Hips** - at the level of the hip joint or the largest circumference of your hips.

9. **Thighs** - At the largest part of each leg measured separately.

10. **Calves** - At the largest part of your calf.

11. **Your weight**. - In pounds or Kilograms.

You can either measure both of the arms and add them together and both of the legs then add them together (which will be more accurate) or just pick one of each and stick with it. (Which is quicker to do).

Measure each part of your body and note it down on the table. Use either centimetres or inches as you prefer – but keep to the same throughout the diet.

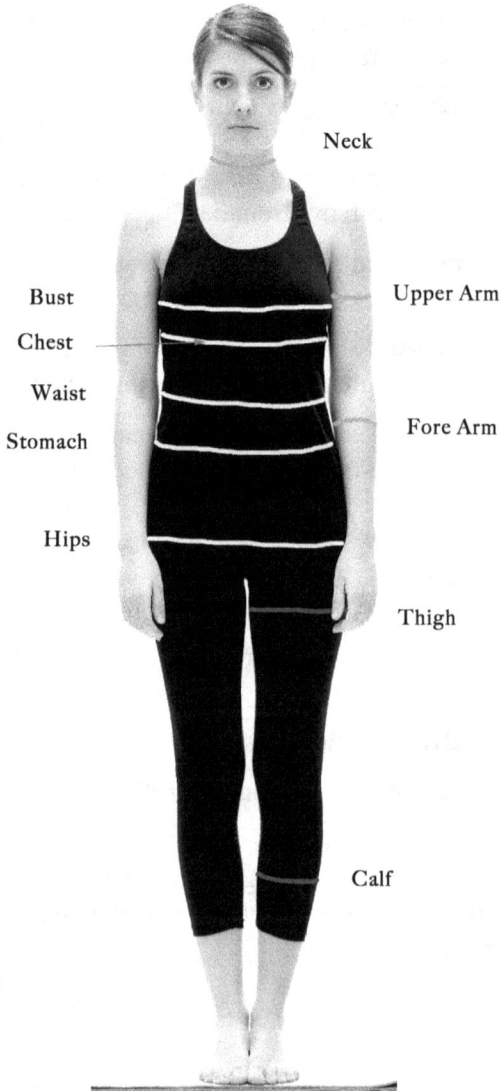

Neck

Bust

Chest

Waist

Stomach

Hips

Upper Arm

Fore Arm

Thigh

Calf

YOUR PROGRESS LOGS

	First Day	End of Week 1	End of Week 2	End of Week 3	End of Week 5	Goal
Neck						
Chest						
Bust						
Upper Arm						
Forearm						
Waist						
Stomach						
Hips						
Thigh						
Calf						
Total for Week						
Weight						

Notes:

20. YOUR HIDDEN STRENGTHS

Without a doubt, one of the best things you can do for yourself is to convince your mind that this diet really is what you want to do. If you dieted and failed before then your mind is going to view this new diet as just a passing fad and 'it' won't take you seriously. If you're doing your first diet, then this will be something even more strange for your mind to cope with as it's unknown territory for it. And it does not like it.

That's why getting your mind on your side is just so important.

I've found one of the most powerful way to do that is to give myself enough excellent reasons why something should be accomplished and made sure to overcome as many objections to doing something as I can. Clearing the path as it were - to make the way forward easier to go along.

Most, if not all diet experts seem to design a diet as purely a process that deals with the physical body. That's as daft designing a car but forgetting it needs a driver in order to make it go where you want it to go. And if the driver is not in control of the car then it will soon go off the road and crash.

Most of the time, your mind will be guiding you in the things you do - it will be in control. And like when you drive a car, much of what you do throughout the day will be on automatic

- you won't even be aware of those little decisions that you are making unconsciously. Another way of putting it is that a lot of what we do throughout the day is done by habit. And habits by their very nature are most always ingrained, deeply ingrained.

But leaving those habitual, unconscious decisions to their own devices, is one easy way to sabotage your fitness and fat loss goals. One truly effective way to overcome those deeply ingrained habits is by training your mind to react in a way that is in keeping with what you have consciously decided to achieve.

This is not a complicated process.

All you need to do is find out what those habits are influencing you to do. Then decide what has to be done in order to retrain them to conform to what you have consciously decided are your wants and desires - or goals in other words.

We looked at this briefly in part one, so now we are going to get down to the nitty gritty of making this process work for you.

Frankly, this need not take very long. Completing these simple step by step exercises will be the difference between you failing or succeeding in your fitness goals.

Your success is in your hands - no one else's.

Here are the tools - you just have to use them! But first a little story to illustrate a point...

21. Overcome Life Stoppers

Step Two

There are so many things that being fat keeps from us. The things we miss out on can range from the simple things like not being able to run around with the children - to missing out on a well earned promotion - to seeing the love of our life going off with some one else.

Yet it seems sad to me that so many people who are carrying just that too much fat don't want to admit to themselves that in fact being over fat does not just hurt us physically - it damages us in so many other ways as well.

Many years ago, I knew a really super guy who I will call Jerry. Jerry was a really sound person and would help any one any way he could. He was bright, intelligent, interesting and on that level would have made a fine catch for any woman of his age and I am certain he would have become loyal husband and a devoted father.

But Jerry was -there is no other way to put it - extremely fat.

Jerry was also at the time young and surprisingly handsome too and he had a eye for the pretty girls whom he could charm with his personality. The sad thing is, he never could develop a long term relationship with them and many times you would see him downcast because once again, the love of his life had moved on.

When you asked the girls he had loved why it didn't work out the they would say that Jerry was a super guy - really he was. But... they could not cope with his size.

Forty years later, Jerry is still single, still living on his own and has never know the joys of lasting love, fatherhood and family life. Being fat caused him to miss out on so much.

But the real question here is 'what have you missed out on?'

You may not have missed out on as much as Jerry but even one thing you didn't have or could not do - was one thing too many.

Take some time to honestly look at your life and see all the things you have missed out on and write them down.

Whatever you do, don't be a Jerry.

Take time now to recognise that carrying around too much fat has slowed you down - not just physically but in many other ways too.

It takes strength and courage to admit when things aren't totally right.

I know that you can find within yourself the strength you need to move on - and through seeing what you may have already missed out on - you'll come to understand just how much you have to gain.

This is an important first step simply because it will serve to highlight - at a very deep level - which way your current habits are steering you.

Once you understand that - you'll be able to use that knowledge to overcome your 'bad' habits and retrain your mind to work with you in a positive and congruent way.

So what have you missed out on?

Let me again give you a few ideas to be going on with ...

- I can't run around with the children/grandchildren.
- I can't go to the beach because people laugh at me.
- I can't take the dog for a walk, it's just too exhausting.
- I can't wear my favourite clothes any more.
- I have so little energy.
- I've been passed over at work because of 'health' problems.
- My love life isn't as good as it used to be.

Now fill in the form on the next page - honestly - and then move on to the next task designed to help you become the person you want to be in the next chapter 'LIST ONE'.

The Things Being Over Fat Kept From Me

1

2

3

4

5

6

7

8

9

10

The Things Being Over Fat Kept From Me

11

12

13

14

15

16

17

18

19

20

The Things Being Over Fat Kept From Me

Notes:

22. LIST ONE
YOUR NEEDS

The Thing I Believe I Need Right Now

This is simply a list of your needs. Those things that a blank cheque from a rich friend could take care of right now. It's important because it could be that some of the things on this list are causing you to be stressed and it may be food has become a comfort for you. OK so that's a simplification. But I'm sure you understand just how these types of problems can affect you.

Don't be afraid about what you put down on this list or limit yourself in any way. Make sure to include anything and everything – even those things you would rather ignore and hope will go away

Some Suggestions...

- All my bills paid.

- Being fit enough to walk the dog.

- Enough money to pay my rent or mortgage and general day-to-day expenses.

- Having the energy to play with the children/ grandchildren.

- Enough income to afford the holiday that I really need to take.

- Being healthy enough to give up the medication I am taking.

- Now you fill in **your** reasons in the form over.

161

List One - The Thing I believe I Need Right Now

1 _____

2 _____

3 _____

4 _____

5 _____

6 _____

7 _____

8 _____

9 _____

10 _____

List One - The Thing I believe I Need Right Now

11

12

13

14

15

16

17

18

19

20

The Thing I believe I Need Right Now

Notes

23. LIST TWO
YOUR WANTS

The Things I Want...

Like I said earlier, it's not just our needs that can make us look to find solace elsewhere. Our wants can also be responsible for unhappiness too - due to an undercurrent of feeling unfulfilled.

Remember its nearly always better to try and do something and fail rather than never have tried at all. Failing only shows you how something does not work – it does not mean you can never succeed – you just have to have faith in yourself and keep trying.

Anyway, this list is all about the things you want whether you need them or not! And don't hold back – let your imagination go wild. Here are some suggestions to get you started...

- Excellent health
- A luxury house
- A million in the bank
- Be super fit
- A happy home life
- Brilliant holidays in exotic places
- Canoeing down the Amazon
- A holiday home in Barbados or _____ fill in the blank.

Turn over to the next page and write out your own list...

165

List Two - The Things I Want...

1

2

3

4

5

6

7

8

9

10

LIST TWO

List Two - The Things I Want...

11

12

13

14

15

16

17

18

19

20

167

The Things I Want...

Notes

24. LIST THREE
PERSONAL TRAITS AND QUALITIES

Personal Traits & Qualities I Want or Need

When you start to think about the things you want and need then it becomes obvious that there is more to life than mere things. While having nice 'stuff' can be good... It is a sad person who thinks that life is made up of just the things they possess.

Here's your chance to include the personal traits and qualities that you think are important for a successful, high quality life.

If you look at the lives of any successful person you'll notice that they all have qualities or attributes of both personality and character in common. Many times we do actually possess those qualities and attributes ourselves, but they remain hidden. And sometimes another persona emerges instead of the real us. That can be down to upbringing, education, peer pressure and who we mix with at work and elsewhere.

The thing is, is that if we keep on doing the same things we are going to get the same results. If you keep banging your head on the wall it's still going to hurt no matter how many time you try it. Virtually without fail - the same actions reap the same rewards.

169

In a nutshell. If you want to change who and what you are - you have to change what you do - it really is that simple.

So if your actually reading this bit and have been filling the forms well done you! That will most probably mean the difference between success and failure. I'd like to congratulate you personally for that so drop me an email to page170@SnackBoxDiet.com

I'd love to hear from you. As I'm certain you will be one of the few whose efforts will be rewarded with success.

One reason why so many people don't succeed on diets is that they are not totally committed to the change in their lives that getting fit will bring - simply because...

People often fear change.

Our attitude towards change is skewed because, many times, the big changes in our lives have been those which have been forced on us - like going to school, moving when our parents changed jobs and that type of thing.

But when it's us who decide on the changes we make then 'change' can and will take on a totally different and wholly positive perspective. Simply because we have taken charge of that change and so have taken charge of our lives.

Enough of that...

I think the list of suggestions will actually help to explain this more readily.

Some suggestions of qualities and characteristics you might want to have...

- Be more disciplined
- Be in good health
- Have a better disposition
- Be friendlier to those around me
- Be enthusiastic
- Be more assertive
- Have real self-confidence
- Believe in myself
- Stop wasting time
- Finish what I start – no matter what
- Enjoy Life to the full

Again, don't censor yourself - if there is a personal quality or trait you like to possess put it down now - matter how odd or stupid you think it may sound to someone else. Their opinion does not matter here as they are not living your life - you are!

Now go to the next pages and fill in the forms listing all the new personal traits and qualities you would like to have

List Three - Personal Traits & Qualities I Want or Need

1

2

3

4

5

6

7

8

9

10

LIST THREE

List Three - Personal Traits & Qualities I Want or Need

11

12

13

14

15

16

17

18

19

20

173

So well done! You have now completed the second most important step on the way to a new You. Now go back to the chapter 'Don't compare yourself to others"

25. Shopping Lists

In an effort to make following this diet as easy as possible, shopping lists for each of the first five weeks have been prepared for you.

They list all the ingredients for each week but obviously I assume you have things like salt and pepper already at home - so they won't be on the list.

Also, to save buying so many things in very small quantities you'll notice that many of the main ingredients are used a number of days running. That does mean you can buy the bigger packs and save some money. It also means that some ingredients will carry over from one week to the next - so do use common sense when buying and check the menu for Monday and Tuesday of the following week too.

By the way. RTE = Ready to Eat.

Shopping List Week One

Meat
Bacon 350g
Chicken Breast 300g RTE
Ham sliced 450g
Roast Beef Slices 150g
Turkey Breast x 2
Turkey Drumsticks x 3 RTE

Fish
Crab Meat RTE 150g
Smoked Salmon 225g RTE
Tuna in Brine 100g

Cheeses
Stilton 50g
Double Gloucester 100g
Goats 50g
Gouda 75g
Hard Parmesan 30g
Leerdammer 50g
Leicester 75g
Mimolette 75g
Monterey Jack 100g
Muenster 50g
Petit Suisse 150g
Port Salut 50g
Quark 50g
Rebluchon 50g
Romano 50g
Shropshire Blue 50g
Swiss 75g
Wensleydale 50g

Salads
Garlic 1
Avocado small 1
Beet root 50g
Carrot Grated 100g
Celery stick 3
Chives 250g
Cucumber 50g
Dill Pickles 4
Green Pepper 1
Lettuce 500g
Mushrooms medm 6
Mustard and Cress 50g
Olives Black 20
Onion 75g
Radishes 12
Red Pepper 1
Romaine 100g
Spring Onion 1
Tomatoes cherry 6
Tomatoes Small 2
Tomatoes Sun Dried 50g
Water Cress 25g
Parsley 5g

Vegetables
Broccoli 40g
Fennel 5 bulbs
Peas 75g
White Cabbage   25g

Nuts and Seeds
Sesame seed 50g
Almonds 50g
Brazil 50g
Cashew 50g
Coconut flesh 100g
Macadamia 50g
Sunflower kernels 25g
Walnuts 50g

Fruit
Apple 3
Tangerine 1
Raisins 30g
Apricot 1
Lemon 1

Dairy
Fromage Blanche 200g
Natural Yogurt 17 pots
Greek Yogurt 2 pot
Soured Cream 30 ml
Pots are 125g size

Extras
Orange juice 15ml
White wine Vinegar 30 ml
Tarragon Vinegar 10ml
Tarragon 2 g
Dill Chopped 30g
Cayenne pepper 1

Ready Mades
Mayo 60 ml
Lemon Juice 100 ml

Peanut Oil 1 ltr
Olive Oil 1 ltr
Sesame Seed Oil 250ml
Honey 250g
Dijon Mustard 200g

Notes:
The quantities given are for
ONE person only.

RTE = Ready To Eat - if you
don't want to cook them
yourself.

If you don't want to buy so
many varieties of cheese - you
can get more of fewer varieties
if you prefer.
You can also get a bag of
mixed salad if you prefer that
to getting individual types of
greens.
For everything else -
obviously some quantities on
the list may be less than the
smallest packet you can buy -
Just get the smallest available
and anyway, things like herbs,
spices and that sort of thing
will probably be used in the
next week or two.

Shopping List Week Two

Meats
Roast Beef Slices 300g
Turkey Breast Grilled 1
Pork/Danish Salami 300g
Chicken Slices 150g
Pepperoni Sausage 300g
Duck Breast RTE 450g
Roasted Lamb Sliced 150g
Pork Tenderloin 50g

Fish
Tuna in Brine 100g
Tuna in Oil 100g
Sardines in Tomato Sauce 300g
Anchovy Fillet 1
Smoked Haddock 300g

Cheeses
Mimolette 75g
Lancashire 50g
Airedale 50g
Jubilee Blue 50g
Jarlsberg 75g
Beaufort 75g
Cottage or Curd 50g
Mozzarella 100g
Gruyère 50g
Canadian Cheddar 75g
Gorgonzola 50g
Cantal 75g
Dauphin 50g
Emmental 50g
Cheddar 75g
Cheshire 50g
Monastery 50g
Double Worcester 50g
Devon Blue 50g
Fountaineblueau 50g

Salads
Garlic Clove 1
Celery stick 5
Chives 30g
Cucumber 100g
Dill Pickles 3
Green Pepper 1
Lettuce 100g
Mush rooms medium 115g
Olives Black 26
Olives Green 20
Onion 50g
Red Pepper 1
Spring Onion 2
Tomatoes Small 6
Water Cress 100g
Sorrel 100g
Palm Hearts 3
Capers 3g
Endives 100g
Escarole 100g
Alfalfa Sprouts 50g
Dandelion Leaves 100g
Spinach 75g
Pimentos 15g

Vegetables
French Beans   100g
Black Eyed Peas   100g

Nuts and Seeds
Sesame seed   50g
Sunflower kernels   50g
walnuts   15g
Peanuts   50g
Pecans   50g
Pine nuts   50g
Pistachios   50g
Pumpkin Seeds   50g

Dairy
Fromage Blanche   250g
Natural Yogurt   5 pots
Greek Yogurt   2 pots
Egg   3

Extras
White wine Vinegar   15ml
Tarragon Vinegar   5g
Hummus   50g
Balsamic Vinegar   5ml
Cider Vinegar   15ml
Parsley   5g
Fresh Basil   3g
Paprika   3g
Whole grain Mustard   5g
Sugar   2g

Fruit
Apple   2
Blueberries   50g

Fresh Figs   1
Gooseberries   50g

Ready Mades
Mayo   45g
Lemon Juice   10ml
Tomato Ketchup   15g
Italian Salad Dressing   15ml

Notes:
The quantities given are for
ONE person only.

RTE = Ready To Eat - if you
don't want to cook them
yourself.

If you don't want to buy so
many varieties of cheese - you
can get more of fewer varieties
if you prefer.
You can also get a bag of
mixed salad if you prefer that
to getting individual types of
lettuce.
For everything else -
obviously some quantities on
the list my be less than the
smallest packet you can buy -
Just get the smallest available
and anyway, thing like herbs,
spices and that sort of thing
will probably be used in the
next week or two.

Shopping List Week Three

Meats
Chicken Breast RTE 150g
Chicken Leg RTE 6
Prosciutto 200g
Roast Beef Slices 350g
Roasted Lamb Sliced 600g
Turkey Drumsticks RTE 2

Fish
Anchovy Fillet
Cod Dried 100g
Smoked Haddock 75g
Smoked Salmon 225g
Salmon in Brine 150g
Shelled Prawns/Shrimp 50g

Cheese
Airedale 50g
American 75g
Beaufort 75g
Boursin 50g
Caerphilly 75g
Cantal 75g
Cheddar 50g
Cour de Chevre 75g
Derby 50g
Dorset Blue 50g
Feta 75g
Goats - dry 125g
Paneer 50g
Roquefort 50g
Saint Paulin 75g
Wensleydale 125g

White Stilton 50g
Yorkshire Blue 50g

Salads
Alfalfa Sprouts
Avocado small 1
Carrot Grated 50g
Celery stick 4
Chives 15g
Cucumber 50g
Endives 100g
Garlic Clove 1
Green Pepper 100g
Iceberg 100g
Lettuce 200g
Mixed Salad (Bag) 100g
Mush rooms medium 9
Mustard and Cress 50g
Olives Black 20
Olives Green 20
Red Pepper 1
Roquette-Arugula 50g
Spinach 25g
Spring Onion 6
Tomatoes cherry 24
Tomatoes Medium 4
Tomatoes Sun Dried 30g
Water Cress

Vegetables
Sugar snap peas 50g

Nuts and Seeds
almonds 100g

Cashew   50g
coconut flesh   100g
Pecans   50g
walnuts   65g
Fruit
Blueberries   25g
Lemon   1
Lime   1
Plum   1
Tangerine   1

Dairy
Fromage Blanche   375g
Greek Yogurt   1 pot
Natural Yogurt   2
Soured Cream   175ml

Extras
Peanut Oil   100ml
Olive Oil   100ml
honey   10g
Dijon Mustard   5g
Balsamic Vinegar   15ml
Cider Vinegar   30ml
Fresh Mint   10g
Herbs de Provance   3g
Lemon Juice   10ml
Orange juice   15ml
Parsley   5g
Plain Flour   15g
Sugar   5g
White wine Vinegar   15ml

Notes:
The quantities given are for

ONE person only.

RTE = Ready To Eat - if you don't want to cook them yourself.

Don't forget to check and see if you do need things like olive oil etc. You may still have plenty left from last week

If you don't want to buy so many varieties of cheese - you can get more in quantity of fewer varieties if you prefer. You can also get a bag of mixed salad if you prefer that to getting individual types of lettuce. There are not too many Vegetables this week so if you want to add some from the OK list - please do...

For everything else - obviously some quantities on the list my be less than the smallest packet you can buy - Just get the smallest available and anyway, thing like herbs, spices and that sort of thing will probably be used in the next week or two.

Shopping List Week Four

Meats

Bacon   100g
Beef Dry Italian   450g
Chicken Leg RTE   4
Chicken Sausages   12
Pate – as you like it   150g
Pork/Danish Salami   100g
Roasted Lamb Sliced
Fillet Steak   125g
Turkey Sausages   18

Fish

Sardines in oil   225g
Smoked Herring   3 fillet
Tuna in Brine   100g

Cheese

Boursin   75g
Brie   75g
Buxton Blue   75g
Camembert   75g
Cheddar   65g
Cottage or Curd   50g
Dauphin   50g
Gouda   75g
Jarlsberg   75g
Lancashire   50g
Leerdammer   50g
Leicester   75g
Mimolette   75g
Monterey Jack   50g
Munster   50g

Petit Suisse   75g
Port Salut   50g
Romano   75g
Roquefort   50g
Saint Paulin   75g
Swiss   75g

Salads

Alfalfa Sprouts   50g
Artichoke hearts   2
Carrot Grated   100g
Celery stick   2
Chives   20g
Cucumber   50g
Endives   100g
Escarole   100g
Green Pepper   1
Iceberg   100g
Lettuce   200g
Mixed Salad (Bag)   300g
Olives Green   20
Onion   65g
Radishes   9
Red Pepper   1
Spinach   100g
Spring Onion   1
Tomatoes cherry   28
Tomatoes Medium   4
Tomatoes Sun Dried   125g
Water Cress   100g

Vegetables

Broccoli   100g

Fennel   1 bulb
White/green Cabbage   50g

Nuts and Seeds
Cashew   15g
Macadamia   50g
Pecans   50g
Peanuts   50g
Pine nuts   50g
Pistachios   50g
Pumpkin Seeds   50g
Sesame seed   50g

Fruit
Apple   2
Lime   1
Peach   1
Raisins   10g
Tangerine   1

Dairy
Fromage Blanche   450g
Egg   1
Greek Yogurt   2 pots
Natural Yogurt   1 pot

Extras
Balsamic Vinegar
Cider Vinegar   30ml
Fresh Basil   3g
Fresh Mint   10g
Fresh Coriander/Cilantro
15g
Lemon Grass   30g
Red wine Vinegar   5ml

Tarragon   3g
Lemon Juice   65ml
Peanut Oil   45ml
Olive Oil   90ml
honey   10g
Dijon Mustard   30g

Ready Made
Mayo   45ml
Sweet chilli Sauce   5ml
Fish Sauce Thai   10ml

Notes:
The quantities given are for
ONE person only.

RTE = Ready To Eat - if you
don't want to cook them
yourself.

If you don't want to buy so
many varieties of cheese - you
can get more of fewer varieties
if you prefer.
You can also get a bag of
mixed salad if you prefer that
to getting individual types of
lettuce.
 Check to make sure you don't
have some stuff already in
stock.

Shopping List Week Five

Meats

Chicken Breast   450g
Chicken Sausages   6
Corned Beef   300g
Ham sliced   150g
Beef Salami   300g
Turkey Drumsticks   3

Fish

Anchovy Fillet   4
Crab Meat RTE   200g
Smoked Salmon   300g
Tuna in Brine   225g

Cheeses

Baby Bel   4
Bath   50g
Canadian Cheddar   75
Cantal   75g
Cheddar   75g
Cheshire   50g
Derby   75g
Devon Blue   50g
Dorset Blue   50g
Double Gloucester   100g
Double Worcester   50g
Emmental   50g
Grafton Village Cheddar   75g
Gruyère   50
Mimolette   75g
Monastery   50
Pepper Jack   50g

Rebluchon   50g
Tomme   75g
Tomme de Chevre   75g
Truffe   50g

Salads

Beet root   50g
Capers   15g
Carrot Grated   50g
Celery stick   3
Chives   25g
Cucumber   1
Dill Pickles   7
Endives   100g
Garlic Clove   1
Green Pepper   1
Iceberg   100g
Lettuce   200g
Mixed Salad (Bag)   100g
Mush rooms medium   150g
Mustard and Cress   50g
Olives Black   10
Olives Green   20
Onion White/Red   250g
Radishes   9
Red Pepper   3
Romaine   100g
Roquette-Arugula   100g
Sorrel   100g
Spring Onion   4
Tomatoes Medium   7
Water Cress   150g

184

Vegetables
Fennel   1 bulb
French Beans   50g

Nuts and Seeds
almonds   50g
Brazil   50g
Cashew   50g
coconut flesh   100g
Pecans   15g
Sunflower kernels   50
walnuts   65g

Fruit
Apple   1
Apricot   1
Blueberries   120g
Lemon   1

Dairy
Fromage Blanche   375g
Egg   4
Greek Yogurt   1Pot
Natural Yogurt   3 pots
Soured Cream   75ml
Double Cream   60ml

Extras
Peanut Oil   15ml
Olive Oil   30ml
honey   5g
Dijon Mustard   5g

Cider Vinegar   35ml
Dill Chopped   10g
Nutmeg   3g
Parsley   55g
Lemon Juice   5ml
Dried Origano   5g
Dried Basil   3g
Garlic Powder   3g

Ready Mades
CousCous   100g
Mayo   150ml
Tomato Ketchup   45ml
Pickled Relish   5ml
Salad Cream   5ml

Notes:
The quantities given are for
ONE person only.

RTE = Ready To Eat - if you
don't want to cook them
yourself.

Check to make sure you don't
have some stuff already in
stock. Again, if you want to
cut down on the variety of
cheeses - you can.

Shopping Lists

Notes

26. A FEW EASY EXERCISES

Like I said earlier in the book - Exercise is not an option if you want to lose any significant amount of fat. It really is compulsory.

If you think about it for minute it's obvious. We don't get fat by eating only what our bodies can 'burn' during the day. We only get fat because we eat more than they need.

You already know that active people use more energy so it stands to reason that by becoming more active you are going to encourage your body to make up the difference between what your body needs and what your giving it by consuming the fat it is carrying around.

The best exercises for this consist of short duration 'sets' that make your heart pump and encourages you to breath deeply - expanding your lungs - Which in turn encourage your body to use fat as energy.

This type of exercise is NOT aerobics!

While long duration exercise will use the energy stored in your fat tissue while your exerting yourself. That fat burning process stops when you stop exercising. On the other hand when done correctly, high energy interval training - not only gets you quickly to the point of burning fat for energy - it encourages the body to continue doing so for hours after you have stopped exercising.

This of course is great news for people like us who need to exercise as part of our fat loss program but don't want to spend hours doing so.

This form of exercise is the best for ongoing fat loss but may not be a good place to start if your not used to doing any exercise at all.

So as that may well be the case - I have included a few gentle exercises you can start with below.

Begin at your own pace and move on as you feel you can.

As your condition improves simply do them faster but for no more than two - three minutes each, for each exercise and have a minute of recovery time between each set.

When you first start the exercises, take your time to get the technique right. Then as you get confident, you can increase the speed you do them at.

Also, you should notice that after a week or two you become more flexible and you'll be able to move your body through a greater range of movement. Make sure you take advantage of that to the full and push yourself just that little bit more each time until you regain full movement of every part of your body.

The exercise I have included here are the ones that cause you to use the bigger muscles in your body. That's because bigger muscles need more energy then he smaller ones and so will burn more energy from your bodies fat. And the time taken to get to that fat burning point will be shorter too, so you don't need to exercise so long to get the same effect.

Here's one last reminder to clear exercise with your medical advisor if you believe that is necessary.

Anyway, on with the exercises.

The Exercises

Hip flexor.

This strengthens the thigh and the hip muscles.

Using the back of a chair or a table for support, stand sideways behind the support, using one hand to balance yourself.

Breathe in and then breathe out slowly as you take five seconds to raise your right leg up at the front, bending the knee as far as you can go.

Hold it for the count of one, then take 3-5 seconds to lower it back down again as you finish breathing out.

Rest for one breath.

Repeat as many times as you can in 1 to 2 minutes, then change legs.

Hip extension.

This is useful to strengthen the lower back muscles as well as the buttocks.

Using the back of a chair or table for support, bend slightly forward at the hips until your body is at about a 45° angle. Breathe in and then breathe out slowly as you put your weight onto your right leg, keep your left leg straight as you take five seconds to slowly lift it out behind you, without bending your knee or your upper body or pointing your toes.

The idea is to try and keep tension on the back of the leg. Once you've got it as far as you can, hold it there for one second, then take 3-5 seconds to lower the leg back down to the starting position as you finish exhaling. Rest for one breath.

Repeat As many times as you can in 1 to 2 minutes then change legs.

Side leg raise.

This strengthens the muscles at the side of your legs and hips.

Again using the back of a chair or table for support, stand upright with your feet slightly apart.

Breathe in and then breathe out slowly as you take five seconds to move your right leg up to the right side with the foot & toes still pointing forwards.

Hold that position for two seconds, then slowly lower your leg back to the standing position as you finish your exhaling.

Rest for one breath.

Repeat As many times as you can in 1 to 2 minutes then change legs.

Knee extension.

This is designed to strengthen muscles in the front of your thighs and shins.

Using a small cushion, place the small cushion at the front of a kitchen chair, sit down on top of it so that the cushion extends to just under your knees. That way, the balls of your feet should be the only part of your foot that's on the ground.

Starting with your right leg, take a deep breath in and as you breathe out, slowly lift your right foot out in front of you, keeping your toes pointed towards the ceiling. Hold it for a count of two, then lower your right leg back down again so that the balls of your feet are touching the floor once more as you finish exhaling.

Repeat As many times as you can in 1 to 2 minutes then change legs.

Take a short pause, repeat again with the right leg as many times as you can and then with the left leg as many times as you can.

Leg Raise

Placing something comfortable on the floor, like a bed cover folded a few times, lay down on the floor on your back. Place your arms on the floor by your side to give you a bit of support.

Bending your legs at the knee, bring your feet up towards your backside. Starting with the right leg, keeping the knee in the same position, gradually lift the lower part of the right leg up until it points about 45°, then keeping the leg straight, continue to lift the whole leg, bringing it over towards your head as far as you can, to the count of 3. Hold it there for one second, then keeping it straight, lower it down to nearly touch the floor again, breathing out as you do.

Take a deep breath in, then breathe out. Repeat raising the straight leg again as far as you can, then lowering it back down nearly to the floor again.

Rest for one breath.

Repeat As many times as you can in 2 to 3 minutes then change legs.

Chair Stand

The first exercise is designed to strengthen primarily the muscles in the abdomen, but will also work to a certain extent on the thighs as well. Using the same kitchen chair, sit to the front of the chair, and lean back so that you are in a half-reclining position, with your back and shoulders straight, but with your knees bent and your feet flat on the floor. You may wish to use a pillow in order to keep your back straight and provide a bit more comfort!

Slowly sit forward – without using your hands (or as little as possible if you must use them), keeping your back straight and bending only at the waist. You should be able to feel it's your stomach muscles that are doing the work. Keep moving forward until you reach the balance point, so that you can stand up, again using your hands as little as possible. Once you've got to the standing position, reverse the process – sit down, and then lean back until your weight is supported by the back of the chair. Take a breath before you start and breathe out as you sit up and finish breathing out as you come back down again.

Take a rest for one breath, then repeat for another 10-15 times.

Professional Help

Now it may be that you would prefer the help of a professional to provide some guidance in how you should exercise. If that is the case, have a look at the contacts I have included at the back of the book.

27. SUPPLEMENTS

The question of supplementation often arises when discussing diet plans.

Simply put, it doesn't matter what diet plan you choose - even - if you were to eat a totally conventional diet - you would still need to take supplements of some kind or another.

The reason for that is simple in that under modern farming and food production methods, foods are no longer grown on nutritionally rich soils or produced from nutritionally rich ingredients. Studies show that the amount of available vitamins and minerals in soil has dropped by over 80% over the last 80 or so years.

So whether you are eating a conventional diet or whether you are on Snack Box or any other diet, you do need to take supplements.

What type of supplements should you take?

Well, that's a very good question.

There are a whole host of supplements available on the market today ranging from a very cheap right up to the ridiculously expensive kind. And to a certain extent you do pay for what you get. But even the most expensive supplements don't deliver as much of the vitamins and minerals that your body needs as they may say they do on the label.

The reason is that for most of these products scientists have isolated the chemical formula that make up the vitamins and have made copies of them from chemicals. They have called these copies say vitamin C or vitamin E or vitamin whatever.

While the chemical formulas for those vitamins may closely resemble that found in nature - it doesn't necessarily mean that if you take 500 mg of the chemical based vitamin C, for instance, that your body will absorb 500 mg of vitamin C.

That's because in nature something like vitamins C is delivered in a package. The package might be an orange or an apple, or something of that type. And it is delivered along with nutrients or trace elements that help the vitamins to be absorbed by your body.

While we have looked at vitamin C here - it is the same for virtually every other vitamin, mineral or trace element you could care to mention.

The bottom line is that you need to try and get your vitamins and minerals in the most natural form possible. Obviously eating food that has been produced in the most natural way using organic methods would be the ideal way of getting the vitamins, minerals and trace elements you need. But for most of us that's going to be virtually impossible which means that we need to rely on taking some sort of supplement or another.

The best are those that are produced from natural ingredients but even there much of the natural potency is lost through the manufacturing process.

The type of multivitamin you will eventually end up taking depends on your own personal taste and finances.

Personally, I think that when you get beyond a certain price point you are most likely paying for a brand name and various levels of commission that go to the people who sold it to you.

So my advice is to pick a mid range supplement that provides a full range of vitamins, minerals and trace elements that your body needs in order to work effectively - and stick with that.

And as the selection of supplements on the market changes so often it's pointless me mentioning a particular brand or type here. But do have a look on the snack box diet website as I may have found one that I can recommend with a clear conscience by the time you read this.

So just to reiterate...

Yes, you do need to take vitamin, mineral and trace element supplements but don't buy the cheapest ones you can find. Neither be impressed by the high-priced brands as I don't believe they will give you any more than you can get with good quality mid-range, mid-priced products.

See www.SnackBoxDiet.com

United States

IDEA Health & Fitness Association

10455 Pacific Centre Court

San Diego, CA 92121-4339

Phone: 800.999.4332, ext. 7

Fax: 858.535.8234

Outside the U.S. and Canada:

Phone: 858.535.8979, ext. 7

Email: contact@ideafit.com

http://www.ideafit.com

Aerobics and Fitness Association of America

15250 Ventura Blvd.,

Suite 200,

Sherman Oaks,

CA 91403.

Phone: 1-877-YOUR-BODY (1-877-968-7263)

Mon-Fri 6:30am-6:30pm Sat 7am-1pm PST

email: see contact form on website

http://www.afaa.com/

The NFTA, The Natural Fitness Trainers Association

P.O. Box 49874, Athens, GA 30606-9998.

Phone 1-(706)623-3671. Weekdays, 11AM-4PM, EST.

email: Contact form on website

http://www. naturalfitnesstrainers.com

Canada

Many of the trainers associations are province based so you'll need to contact them directly.

If you want up to find a trainer near you- you will find the local school or collage a good place to start. Otherwise see…

Can-Fit-Pro

110-255 Consumers Road

Toronto, ON

M2J 1R4

CANADA

Toll Free (outside of the Greater Toronto Area): 1-800-667-5622

Local (within the GTA): (416) 493-3515

Fax: (416) 493-1756

email: info@canfitpro.com

http://www.canfitpro.com

Certified Professional Trainers Network (CPTN) Inc.

122 D'arcy Street

Toronto, Ontario

M5T 1K3

E-mail Address info@cptn.com

Phone Number (416) 979-1654

Fax Number (416) 979-1466

For more associations see http://www.canadianfitness.net/rescen.html

United Kingdom

National Register of Personal Trainers

NRPT.co.uk

4 Bradbury Road

Newnham

Northants NN11 3HD

Tel no: 0844 8484 644

http://www.nrpt.co.uk

email contact form on website

The Fitness Industry Association (FIA)

Castlewood House

77–91 New Oxford Street

London

WC1A 1PX

Tel: 020 7420 8560

Fax: 020 7420 8561
email:contact form on website

http://www.fia.org.uk

Australia

The ASC is one of the largest state back organisation going. It has a massive website that has so much info you can't actually find what you want.

It is probably best to ring them and ask for the info direct.

Failing that, your local school or collage will be able to point you in the right direction.

Australian Sports Commission

Leverrier Cres,

Bruce

ACT 2617 or

PO Box 176,

Belconnen

ACT 2616

Telephone: +61 02 6214 1111

Facsimile: +61 02 6251 2680

http://www.ausport.gov.au/

New Zealand

REP has the best website we've seen for ease of use and finding a trainer.

NZ Register of Exercise Professionals

PO Box 22-374,

Christchurch,

New Zealand

0800 554 499

(International callers dial +64-3-379-6139) 0800 248 348

(International callers dial +64-3-3777-778)

info@reps.org.nz

http://www.reps.org.nz

Other countries.

Try your local school or college first. Also many youth and community associations have links and contacts.

28. INDEX

Don't forget you can get the latest information on the Snack Box Diet by visiting...

www.SnackBoxDiet.com

There is a special section for owners of the book being planned too.

Other books by Mark Moxom

Guaranteed Diet Success

Easy Exercise for Fat Loss

About the Author

Mark Moxom BEng, MEng is a semi retired engineer. Graduating from the University of Plymouth where he received two degrees in communications and information engineering.

He has built up a substantial amount of knowledge on natural health and diet and is the author of a number of books and articles in this field.

He spends a lot of his time in France and speaks both French and English and easy access to the vast riches of European cultures has given him opportunity to gain a good working insight into international cuisine and diet.

"The most successful people in life are generally those who have the best information."

Benjamin Disraeli

www.ingramcontent.com/pod-product-compliance
Lightning Source LLC
Chambersburg PA
CBHW072218270326
41930CB00010B/1901